The Sardine Diet

The Sardine Diet

Lose Weight, Fight Disease & Stay Healthy for Life

A Complete and Easy Plan
Developed by
Keri Glassman, M.S., R.D., C.D.N.

Til Ulf Jespersen

Copyright © 2006 Downtown Bookworks Inc.

President Julie Merberg
Director Patty Brown
Editor Sara Newberry
Writer Susan Wyler
Design Jon Glick, Mouse+Tiger Design

Special thanks Robert Montano, Gordon Wright, Winston Albert, Kimberly Strub, and Sarah Parvis

ISBN 1-59971-456-6

Notice: The information presented in this book is in no way intended as medical advice or as a substitute for medical counseling. The information should be used in conjunction with the guidance and care of your physician. Consult your physician before beginning this or any weight-loss or weight-maintenance program. The recipes in this book are to be followed exactly as written. Neither the publisher nor the authors are responsible for your specific health or allergy needs that may require medical supervision, or for any adverse reactions to the recipes contained in the book.

CONTENTS

Introduction

In the following pages, you will discover why sardines are a dieter's delight. You will also learn just how important these tasty little fish can be to your overall physical well-being. Most significant, you'll be introduced to the Sardine Diet, a delicious, easy, nutritional plan that capitalizes on sardines' unique properties to help you lose weight *and* improve your health. After just one month of delicious meals, you'll not only look better, you'll feel better, too!

If you're like most Americans, you probably have more than one good reason for changing the way you eat. Whether you're overweight or you suffer from one of the many systemic diseases linked to diet, you've got a lot of company. Close to two-thirds of Americans are now classified as overweight. Of those, almost a third are clinically obese, which means that they are at least 30 percent above the recommended weight for their age, sex, and height.

Being overweight makes people more susceptible to many physical problems, including diabetes, heart disease, high blood pressure, and even cancer. At least one-third of Americans have, or are at risk for, type 2 diabetes. More than 16 million suffer from hypertension, or high blood pressure, and that's just for starters. Asthma, allergies, arthritis, and other autoimmune and inflammatory diseases are on the rise.

Many scientists and doctors blame misguided nutritional information as part of the reason for the rise in these ailments. Changes in lifestyle, stress, and the tempting appeal of convenience and fast foods are also major factors. On top of that, many of us have a genetic predisposition to certain chronic diseases.

There is some good news, however. Scientific studies have shown time and again that what you eat can make an enormous difference in your health and in your quality of life. A diet based on the proper nutrients—vitamins, minerals, omega-3 fatty acids, and lean protein—can actually combat some of the laundry list of ills mentioned above. With the right balance of calories and fat and plenty of fiber, such a diet can also help you lose weight painlessly. The best news is that this diet has already been developed for you. To learn more about it, read on.

The Sardine Diet is really a "fishy" name for a high-fiber, reduced-calorie diet that's high in omega-3 fatty acids (more on these in a bit). It actually involves eating a wide variety of foods. Sardines simply make it easy to follow, even on a hectic schedule. Plus, sardines offer the richest, purest source of omega-3 fatty acids you can find, and it is this vital nutrient that has been found to be most lacking in the average American diet.

Studies have proved that including omega-3s in your diet can raise good cholesterol (HDL) while lowering bad cholesterol (LDL) and triglycerides in the blood. Essential fatty acids also act as antioxidants, keeping cells vital and preventing the formation of damaging free radicals. They even have anticlotting properties that keep blood flowing

Did You Know? A sardine is not one particular species of fish. Almost two dozen species of ocean fish, including herring, pilchard, and sprats, are processed and packaged as "sardines."

smoothly. Omega-3s help to lower blood pressure, and they function as an important anti-inflammatory agent. You could think of the omega-3s as a sort of dietary aspirin.

Perhaps most surprising, these oils actually help burn off fat when they are included in meals in the right amounts. For all these reasons, essential fatty acids are often referred to as "good fats." Later on in this book, you'll learn about the most recent scientific studies on how omega-3s improve your health and boost your metabolism, so you'll really understand which foods are good for you and why.

Of course, with the Sardine Diet you'll be eating a lot more than sardines. The detailed Menu Plan, which you'll find on page 46, offers a wide variety of ingredients and flavors, including other lean sources of protein, whole grains, vegetables, nuts, and fruits high in fiber. The diet ensures that you eat all the "good fats," protein, vitamins, and minerals you need. It is also high in calcium, found in leafy greens, almonds, low-fat dairy, and—you guessed it—sardines!

You'll fill up with the right foods—ones that are low in calories and have a low glycemic index. This means that when they're metabolized by the body, they do not quickly raise your blood-sugar level—one of the reasons they help you lose weight and prevent type 2 diabetes. Eating nutrient-rich snacks between meals minimizes the hunger pangs that can lead to binge eating, and since the foods are carefully chosen for maximum benefit and minimum calories, you won't feel hungry or deprived.

Did You Know?

Sardines are one of the most convenient foods for people on the run.

Sardines are extremely popular for desktop lunches, because to eat them all you need to do is flip open the can. The best sardines are now packed in an assortment of flavors, including mustard sauce, tomato sauce, salsa, and pesto. The classic plain varieties come lightly smoked or packed in spring water, soy oil, or olive oil. Many people top sardines with a splash of lemon (the traditional accompaniment to fish), a slice of sweet onion, or a small dollop of mustard or low-fat mayonnaise. They are great over salads, cottage cheese, or pasta. For more ways to enjoy sardines, see the recipes on pages 60 to 127.

You'll also learn how vital calcium and vitamin D are to your body, why they must be consumed in combination, and why sardines are among the best natural sources of these nutrients. The importance of other vital elements, such as vitamin C, folic acid, and trace minerals, will be examined as well.

The Sardine Diet presents a superb and sustainable nutritional plan that's simple to follow and designed to improve your overall health while melting away excess pounds. To make the diet supereasy and painless to follow, we've included a whole month's worth of detailed menus, including three meals a day plus two snacks that you get to choose–all made up of foods that are simple to prepare and satisfying to eat.

So read on to learn all about the goodness, as well as good taste, of sardines. Understanding in detail how diet in general and omega-3 fatty acids in particular affect your health may well be the final incentive you need to give yourself the most valuable gift of all–a slimmer, revitalized you and a better way of eating for the rest of your life.

Chapter One:

Why We Need to Change the Way We Eat

The two most obvious reasons for making a change in your diet—are *weight* and *health.* Sardines target both these concerns, making them a true "superfood." What's more, they're low in calories and packed with protein—and incredibly easy to incorporate into any eating plan.

Dieting to Lose Weight

If you are overweight and don't like the way you look and feel, finding the right diet and sticking to it can pose a tremendous challenge. As most people are well aware, losing weight is not just a cosmetic issue; it is vital to your health.

Being even slightly overweight increases your risk of developing "metabolic syndrome," a disorder that includes high blood pressure, high cholesterol, and high blood-sugar levels, physiological malfunctions that can lead to type 2 diabetes. A large-scale study by the Johns Hopkins Bloomberg School of Public Health found a direct correlation between obesity and type 2 diabetes. Being overweight raises blood pressure and puts a strain on all your major organs. Obesity is literally a heartbreaking condition. Chronic obesity has been scientifically linked to a host of systemic ailments, especially inflammatory and autoimmune diseases. It can also lead to painful psychosocial issues, as well as sleep apnea and orthopedic problems.

Most people are overweight because they eat too much and their diet is nutritionally out of balance. Most of us do not get enough exercise. Just looking at that bike won't do it.

What Does It Mean to Be Overweight?

The Centers for Disease Control and Prevention, a division of the United States Department of Health and Human Services, defines "overweight" as a body mass index (BMI) of greater than 25. Anyone with a BMI of 30 or higher is classified as obese. A BMI of 18.5 to 24.9 is considered normal; below that is underweight.

There is a simple formula for determining your body mass index:

$$\text{BMI} = \frac{\text{Your weight in pounds}}{\text{Your height in inches squared}} \times 703$$

For example, a woman who is 5′2″ and weighs 125 pounds would calculate her BMI as follows:

5′2″ = 62 inches

62 X 62 = 3,844

125 ÷ 3,844 = .0325

.0325 X 703 = BMI of 22.84

Another indication of obesity is a waist greater than 40 inches for men and 35 inches for women. Waist-to-hip ratio is also a valuable tool in estimating health status. Calculate the waist-to-hip ratio by dividing the waist circumference by the hip circumference. It is important because body fat located in the upper body (especially abdominal region) can be risky in terms of one's health profile. For women, a waist-to-hip ratio of 0.8 or lower is considered healthy; for men, it's 0.95 or lower.

Much of the obesity problem in America is due to our diet, which includes too much fast food. We eat far too many saturated and trans-fats and refined carbohydrates, as well as not enough healthful fruits and vegetables, especially green leafy vegetables, good fats, and whole grains.

Reducing your BMI—that is, getting your weight under control in proportion to your height and age—will have a huge effect on your health, as well as on how you look and feel. Even if other diets have let you down, you'll find the Sardine Diet easy to follow, easy to incorporate into your busy lifestyle, and extremely effective for many reasons:

1. It addresses the latest, most up-to-date scientific findings on nutrition:

    - Ω Sardines are low in calories and high in lean protein and valuable vitamins and minerals.

    - Ω They are one of the best natural sources of omega-3 fatty acids and calcium paired with vitamin D—all in one package.

2. The diet includes all the major food groups, so your body gets every nutrient it needs, but you don't overeat.

3. Because the Sardine Diet contains so many vegetables, whole grains, fruits, and low-fat dairy products—and because Nordic brisling sardines are so versatile—the meals are full of variety. It is a convenient diet that is never boring, always easy to follow, and delicious to eat.

Did You Know? Nordic brisling sardines are the mildest, most delicate sardines. That's because of the way they are harvested and processed. Only the smallest fully-developed fish with the best flavor, living in deep cold waters, are chosen. Then they are purified, lightly smoked over oak, and packed by hand.

Dieting to Improve Your Health

Doctors and nutritionists have for some time been aware of the critical importance of diet—not only in controlling weight, but in preventing and even curing many chronic illnesses. One big problem with the traditional American diet is the types of fats we eat. In Chapter Two, you'll find a comprehensive guide to good and bad fats, but it's important to note that many doctors believe so-called bad fats are a significant factor in the rise of heart disease and stroke. Many other nutrients are important to your health as well. Among them are:

Calcium. This mineral is essential for building strong teeth and bones. It also plays an important role in the transmission of nerve impulses, muscle contractions, and blood clotting. While other sources of calcium abound—in dairy and leafy greens—those foods lack natural vitamin D, without which calcium cannot be absorbed (milk is fortified with vitamin D). Sardines are not only an excellent source of calcium, but they also contain enough vitamin D to facilitate calcium absorption.

Vitamin D. Very few foods contain significant amounts of vitamin D, but sardines do. Vitamin D is produced in the skin upon exposure to sunlight. Now considered essential to good health, it prevents rickets and acne, and some believe that vitamin D also aids in cancer prevention. A few doctors have even made the radical suggestion that we go outside without sunscreen to be sure we get enough. However, given the rising rates of melanoma (also caused by exposure to the sun's rays), most doctors don't recommend that. Instead, they say, make sure you eat enough sardines and other oily fish—the best natural dietary source of vitamin D. Just two servings a week can make a significant difference in your health.

Vitamin A. While red and orange vegetables are great sources of vitamin A, this vital nutrient is also found in fish oil. Vitamin A is particularly important for eyesight and skin.

Vitamin C. One of the best antioxidants around and an excellent immune-system booster, vitamin C is readily found in citrus fruits as well as in many other fruits and vegetables, like potatoes, cabbage, and tomatoes.

Fiber. Fiber is the indigestible part of plant materials. It is vital to keeping your digestive tract healthy. It keeps you feeling full longer and helps stabilize blood sugar levels. The Sardine Diet offers lots of fiber in whole grains, vegetables, and the right fruits.

Lean Protein. In addition to sardines, this menu plan includes plenty of protein that is low in fat—from other oily fish to salmon, low-fat dairy, tofu, lean chicken and turkey, and legumes.

Omega-3 Fatty Acids. These "good fats," which are hard to come by except in fish oils (they're found in lesser quality in some nuts and green leafy vegetables), are essential to good health. Find out the details in the next chapter.

Chapter Two:

Good Fats/Bad Fats

IN RECENT YEARS, an understanding of the way the body uses fats has changed the nutritional landscape. There is a new awareness that some fats—namely, saturated fats from meat—are bad for you, while others, such as essential fatty acids like omega-3s, are good for you. The concept of good fats vs. bad fats not only prompted the government to revamp the USDA Food Pyramid, it gave nutritionists and dietitians vital new information in their fight against obesity, type 2 diabetes, heart disease, and hypertension.

Many doctors and dietitians believe that the former USDA Food Pyramid inadvertently fueled the obesity epidemic in America, thanks to its emphasis on carbohydrates, which led people to consume far too many calories. In addition, the old pyramid's misleading premise that all fats are bad and should be avoided was dead wrong. It caused people to shy away from a lot of good fats while they often continued to eat high quantities of hidden trans fats. Found in many packaged foods, trans fats increase the shelf life of food and make crackers and many other foods crisp. Most experts now believe that trans fats are the most damaging of all—and because so many packaged foods contain them, they're particularly hard to avoid.

Certain polyunsaturated fats, especially omega-3s and omega-6s, are considered good fats, because they are absolutely necessary to our physical well-being. Like most vitamins, they cannot be synthesized by the body and must be consumed in food. Without them, we could not survive, which is why they are called "essential."

These good fats can actually help lower bad cholesterol (LDL), a fat-like substance that clogs the arteries. Omega-3s, contained in sardines, also tend to raise good cholesterol (HDL) and lower triglycerides. Consuming plenty of omega-3s helps cleanse the arteries, keeping them healthy and free of plaque.

Most significant for dieters is the way omega-3s affect metabolism. All oils contain 120 calories per tablespoon, but, unlike other oils, omega-3s help oxygenate all your tissues and speed up your metabolism, which actually helps you lose weight. Think of it as good fats conquering bad fats. When your metabolism is speeded up, you burn calories more efficiently. Combined with proper diet and exercise, you will eventually melt off those pounds. In addition, omega-3s improve the speed of nerve impulses to the muscles and smooth out mood swings. Some researchers even believe they help alleviate depression.

The government's Food Pyramid has undergone a couple of substantial revisions of late, but most doctors and other nutrition professionals agree that the latest version is too confusing. As a result, many nutritionists are constructing their own nutritional pyramids that offer people simple and effective ways to structure their diets. That's why the Sardine Diet presents its own food pyramid, which advocates a balanced approach to sound nutrition—including plenty of blockbuster omega-3s.

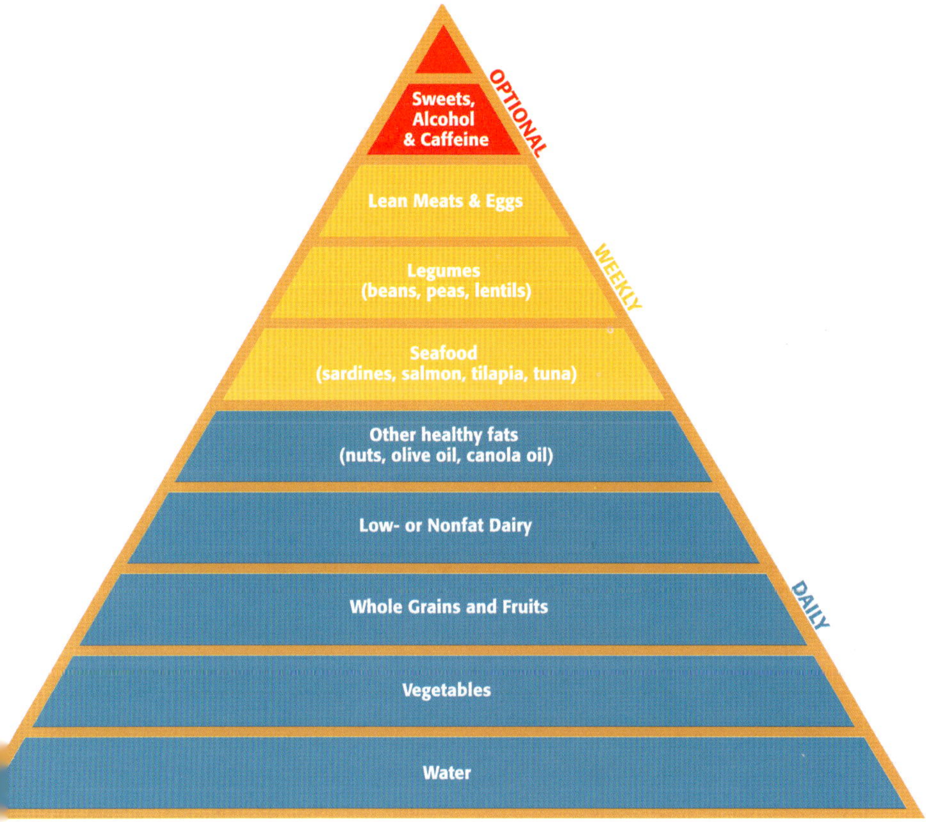

Since the Sardine Diet presents an eating plan that has already screened out bad fats and incorporated good fats for you in the right proportions, what follows is a brief summary of the different kinds of fats you need to be aware of.

What Are the Bad Fats?

- Saturated fats are the ones that are solid at room temperature. They tend to raise bad cholesterol and clog your arteries. They should make up a very small part of your daily diet. Saturated fats are found in meat, butter, and cheese, as well as the oils from a few plants, such as palm and coconut.

- Trans fats are polyunsaturated fats that have been processed so they remain hard at room temperature. They are common in processed foods like crackers, chips, and cookies because they are extremely stable and have a long shelf life. Margarine and shortening are both made up of trans fats. They are particularly damaging because they lower good cholesterol and raise both bad cholesterol and triglycerides, creating the perfect scenario for clogged arteries and heart disease. It's very important to read labels, because any number of packaged foods you might think of as low in fat may actually contain large quantities of trans fats.

What Are the Good Fats?

- Unsaturated fats are liquid at room temperature. Some unsaturated fats actually help lower bad cholesterol (LDL) and raise good cholesterol (HDL). Most vegetable oils are unsaturated. So are fish oils. But not all unsaturated fats are alike, and some, like the oils in sardines, are much more beneficial than others. There are two general categories of unsaturated fats: monounsaturated and polyunsaturated.

- Monounsaturated fats are very stable and have antioxidant properties that prevent the formation of free radicals, dangerous molecules that can cause cancer. Extra-virgin olive oil and canola oil are monounsaturated oils; avocados also are a good source. When used in place of saturated fats, these good fats can lead to a reduction of bad cholesterol and an increase in good cholesterol. Many experts speculate that the good health of people who live in Mediterranean countries has a lot to do with their regular use of olive oil, as well as the prevalence of fish and vegetables in their diet—just like in the Sardine Diet.

Ω Polyunsaturated fats are liquid at room temperature and include fish oils and most vegetable oils, including corn oil, peanut oil, and safflower oil. For years, studies looking at the health benefits of polyunsaturated fats were inconclusive. That's because these oils were all lumped together. Most vegetable oils are high in omega-6 fatty acids, while fish oil is a rich source of omega-3 fatty acids. When studies examined the difference between these two fats, the results were startling.

While our bodies need some omega-6s, in large doses they can be inflammatory and damaging to the body. But omega-3s are anti-inflammatory and extremely beneficial to good health in many ways. The trick is to eat the right balance of these two fatty acids, and that's what you get in the Sardine Diet.

Essential fatty acids, like omega-3s, which are a kind of extra-liquid polyunsaturated fat, are the most valuable fats in the human diet. Your body needs these fats, or lipids, to create a whole range of processes that allow it to function properly, prevent illness, and heal itself. In fact, no person could survive without these fats. That's why they are called "essential."

Your brain is largely made up of fat, and your neurological system needs certain oils, such as omega-3s, which are found

The Essential Balancing Act

As we just learned, there are two kinds of essential fatty acids: omega-3s and omega-6s. It turns out that the average American diet contains way too much omega-6, because that particular type of oil is abundant in meat, shellfish, eggs, and many vegetable oils. But few of us get enough omega-3 oils. Sardines, other oily fish, and certain seaweeds are the only foods that offer them in their most valuable and useful forms.

Because omega-6 and omega-3 oils are processed through some of the same pathways in the body, too much omega-6 actually interferes with the benefits of the omega-3s. That's why you need to eat meals that contain these fats in the right proportions. Calculating this yourself would be a daunting task, much harder than counting calories or carbs. But the Sardine Diet has already done the legwork for you. It contains both of these essential oils in the ratios you need to maximize their health benefits and help you lose weight.

solely in the fish oil in sardines and other oily fish—and in a lesser form in flaxseeds, pumpkin seeds, sunflower seeds, walnuts, and leafy green vegetables—to work at peak performance, avoid depression, and stimulate neural signals. Maybe that's why our grandparents and great-grandparents called fish "brain food."

These essential oils also help muscles contract. Most important for many people, omega-3 fatty acids, like the kind found in sardines, keep blood vessels limber and enhance the free flow of blood, reducing the chances of clots and strokes.

Lowest Mercury Levels

¤ Clams
¤ Oysters
Shrimp
Tilapia
Sardines
Crawfish
Haddock
Trout (freshwater)
‡ Herring
Catfish
Flatfish (includes flounder and sole)
Mackerel (Atlantic)
Scallops
Crab (blue, king, and snow)
Pollock
Shad (American)
Squid
Tuna (canned chunk light)
Lobster (spiny)
Mackerel Chub (Pacific)
• Cod
Perch (freshwater)
Skate
Halibut
Mackerel-Spanish (S. Atlantic)
• Monkfish
• Snapper
Weakfish (sea trout)
Bass (saltwater; includes sea bass/striped bass/rockfish)
Lobster (Northern/American)
‡ Bluefish
Tuna (canned, white albacore)
Tuna (fresh/frozen)
Mackerel-Spanish (Gulf of Mexico)
Marlin
• Orange Roughy
• Grouper
Salmon-canned Pacific (2 servings/week)
‡ -wild Pacific, fresh/frozen (2 servings/month)
‡ -farmed/Atlantic, fresh/frozen (1 serving every 2 months)
Mackerel-King (Atlantic & Gulf of Mexico)
• Shark
• Swordfish
• Tilefish (Gulf of Mexico)

Highest Mercury Levels

KEY

‡ contains PCBs or other pollutants

¤ rarely tested for mercury

• overfished

What about the Extra Oil?

If you're worried that all this extra oil will cause weight gain, fear not. On the Sardine Diet, you'll reduce your total fat intake and eat fewer calories than before. Studies have shown that, in terms of losing weight, the bottom line with any diet is calories. Even diets that claim to work for unusual reasons—food pairing or blood type, for example—actually reduce the total number of calories you ingest. It's simple: Weight comes off every time you expend more calories than you take in. That's one reason exercise helps, too.

Some of the most intriguing evidence of the health potential of omega-3s was discovered a couple of years ago during a study of the native Inuit people of Greenland. These hunters, who traditionally roamed territories above the Arctic Circle and lived almost exclusively on a diet of fish from the ocean and wild animals, ate a diet exceptionally high in fat. Yet these people showed no signs of heart disease, stroke, arteriosclerosis (hardening of the arteries), or atherosclerosis (buildup of plaque on the arterial walls).

Why Are the Fish Oils from Sardines So Beneficial?

Fish oils provide the best natural way by far to obtain omega-3 fatty acids. Nordic brisling sardines from clean, cold, northern fjords offer a concentrated source of these essential oils. They are also free of the chemicals often found in farmed fish and don't pose the same risk of mercury or PCB toxicity—an increasingly common concern in larger ocean fish.

Did You Know?

People who eat sardines or other fish two or more times a week reduce the chance of sudden death from heart attack and stroke by at least 50 percent. There is some discussion about how much of this benefit comes from avoiding saturated fats and how much is due to our consumption of omega-3s, but the fact has been substantiated by numerous studies. The American Heart Association recommends that we should eat omega-3 fatty acids from fish to protect our hearts. For middle-aged and older men, as well as postmenopausal women, the benefits of eating fish far outweigh the risks of mercury within the established guidelines. In October 2005, the Harvard Center for Risk Analysis released a study confirming that, for men and women, decreased fish consumption leads to an increased incidence of stroke and coronary heart disease.

Scientists eventually concluded that their amazingly good cardiovascular health was attributable to the amount of fish they ate. The preponderance of fat in their diet came from fish and marine mammals and was extremely rich in omega-3s. The same holds true for Japan, where people eat very little saturated fat and a lot of fish—and also have a low incidence of heart disease.

Both of these societies are also distinctive in that, traditionally, obesity wasn't an issue. When these populations altered their diets to include a more Western way of eating, either because of changes in the ecosystem or in the culture, they both put on weight and developed the cardiovascular problems characteristic of Americans.

Good Fat/Bad Fat Recap

- Ω Your body needs fat in order to function properly.
- Ω In general, you want to avoid saturated fats and replace them with polyunsaturated and monounsaturated oils.
- Ω The cardiovascular and neurological systems in particular need certain essential fats.
- Ω The most beneficial are the omega-3 essential fatty acids, which are primarily found in fish oils. Sardines offer the best, purest fish oil in a protein-rich package.
- Ω For a healthy diet, you need to both reduce the amount of omega-6 fatty acids and boost your intake of omega-3s. The Sardine Diet will make this much easier for you.
- Ω When coupled with moderate exercise, the omega-3 fatty acids in fish oil actually help to boost metabolism and help you lose weight.

Chapter Three:

The Sardine Diet

Now that you've absorbed so much information about fats and understand all about the essential fatty acid balancing act, you're ready to begin the Sardine Diet.

It's not only an eating plan carefully tailored to make sure you get that all-important balance of omega-3s and -6s (which is why sardines are so important to the diet); it's also a comprehensive, nutritious plan designed for success. The best, most effective diet is the one you can stay on, and the Sardine Diet is designed to enable you to do just that.

Whether you need to lose five pounds or fifty, it's likely you've tried any number of trendy diets before. Either they didn't work or they were impossible to sustain. So why try again–and why try the Sardine Diet?

One main reason: You deserve to look and feel the best you can, and with this eating plan, reaching that goal will be much easier. Read on and you'll understand why this is not only a diet that will work for you now, but a lifestyle-changing diet that offers nutritional guidance and practical lessons that you can apply long after you've moved beyond the intensive first month.

The Sardine Diet helps you shed excess weight even as it improves your health. It fosters a way of eating that makes you feel so good and offers so much satisfaction that you'll want to continue it even when the weight is gone. That's why we've added an extra "maintenance stage," which offers a way to stay on the plan for as long as you like. It's a diet designed to improve your quality of life.

In addition to addressing a host of health issues, good nutrition affects the way you look and feel. After only a few days on the diet, you'll notice an improvement in your energy level and your ability to concentrate. Two of the biggest complaints of people who seek nutritional advice are fatigue and poor focus—and often they don't realize that those issues are enormously affected by what they eat.

The Sardine Diet is scientifically calibrated to give you all the vital nutrients you need within a reduced-calorie framework that assures weight loss in as little as four weeks. That's one month of healthful eating to slim down, boost your metabolism, and improve your overall health, particularly from a cardiovascular standpoint. The diet is exceptionally effective because it is so comprehensive.

To begin with, the Sardine Diet is rich in four basic types of nutrients:

1) Each daily plan offers **omega-3 essential fatty acids** from sardines and other oily fish, as well as from leafy greens and other vegetables, flaxseeds, and olive oil. It also limits the amount of omega-6s you consume, so you eat an appropriate, healthful balance of 5:1 or less, as recommended by most doctors and registered dietitians.

2) The menus are high in **vitamins, antioxidants, and good fats.** They include plenty of vegetables, especially leafy

greens, so that you get a full complement of vitamins A, C, and E, which offer the best antioxidant protection to your body. Think of antioxidants as natural preservatives. They keep your cells healthy and intact and prevent the formation of free radicals, which are associated with wrinkles, plaque in the arteries, and cancer.

3) It is high in **fiber.** Every single meal, and many snacks, include at least one–and often two or three–high-fiber foods. Every day you get to eat a delicious assortment of fiber-rich vegetables, whole grains, and fruits to improve your health and fill you up, ensuring that you never feel hungry. Both the American Heart Association and the American Cancer Society recommend a high-fiber diet to help prevent heart disease and cancer. Fiber helps move foods through your gastrointestinal system, and it is often credited with lowering cholesterol.

4) The Sardine Diet is rich in **calcium,** a mineral that is vital not only to building strong teeth and bones, but also to proper muscle function (including the heart muscle) and the transmission of nerve impulses. Calcium is vital to the cell regulation of your entire body. A 3.75-ounce serving of Nordic brisling sardines offers more than 20 percent of your daily calcium needs. And since sardines also contain vitamin D, your body absorbs the calcium more efficiently.These two nutrients are grouped together because your body needs vitamin D in order to take up the calcium. One of the two snacks you are encouraged to eat every day is low-fat dairy products or sardines to ensure that you get enough of this vital mineral.

Sardines are one of the few foods that naturally contain a significant amount of both of these nutrients. Milk, a rich source of calcium, has little natural vitamin D. It is artificially fortified with vitamin D to help with calcium absorption, but recent studies have called into question the effectiveness of milk and other dairy products in building and maintaining bone. According to statistics compiled from the Harvard Nurses Study, one of the largest epidemiological studies ever done, drinking three or more glasses of milk per day does nothing to reduce the risk of hip or arm fractures. The study, which followed 78,000 women (34 to 59 years of age) for twelve years beginning in 1980, found that fracture rates were actually higher for women who drank more than three (8-ounce) glasses of milk a day than for those who had no dairy products. This makes calcium-rich foods, like kale, sardines, and broccoli, all the more important.

The Sardine Diet is easy to follow and effective because it also offers the following benefits:

- **Low-calorie/no counting.** The Sardine Diet is a low-calorie diet based on an average of 1,250 calories a day. Follow the menu plans and no counting is needed.
- **Variety.** It encompasses all the major food groups. Those 1,250 calories are spread out in an eating plan that is well balanced in fats, protein, and carbohydrates. By eating all kinds of foods, you are assured of getting the vitamins and minerals you need the old-fashioned way: naturally. Also, portions are carefully controlled where necessary (you can eat all the green vegetables you like), but the diet includes many different foods, with a variety of tastes and textures, so you stay satisfied.

- **Balanced fats.** With the Sardine Diet, you get 30 to 35 percent of your calories from fat, which is a normal percentage. But much of it is from "good fats," especially the valuable omega-3 fatty acids found in sardines and other oily fish. This menu plan also gives you the correct proportion of omega-6 to omega-3 fatty acids, which is essential if your body is to utilize them properly.

- **Freedom of choice.** Snacks are a vital part of the Sardine Diet. You get two a day, and you get to choose them from the list on page 58.

- **Satisfaction.** Because you eat three meals a day plus two snacks, and because the diet is high in fiber and low in foods with a high glycemic index, your blood sugar levels remain stable throughout the day. Good fats impart a feeling of satiety (fullness). You eat often enough so that you don't feel hungry or deprived. And since you're allowed a wide range of foods that taste good, the variety adds to feelings of contentment.

  Filling up is easy, because you are allowed as many green vegetables as you like. Wherever the menu plan lists a vegetable but includes no amount, you can eat as much as you like. That said, it's important to eat until you are just satisfied, not stuffed.

- **Reward.** Not only will the Sardine Diet reward you by making you slimmer, healthier, and more energetic; it has a built-in bonus system. Stick to the diet all week, and reward yourself with any one of a list of sweet treats on Saturday night—or any night you choose.

How to Work the Diet

You are now ready to try the Sardine Diet! Here's how it works. On pages 50–57, you'll find a month's worth of detailed menus. Three complete meals are prescribed every day, along with two snacks: one midmorning and one between lunch and dinner. These menus average 1,250 calories a day. **It is essential that you eat every meal and do not skip snacks.** The quantities and portions are designed to help maintain your blood sugar level, so you avoid getting terribly hungry and craving all kinds of things you shouldn't touch.

Eating regularly discourages binging and teaches good dietary habits that you can use for the rest of your life. In fact, learning which foods are good for you, how to balance your menus, and when to eat throughout the day are important lessons for winning the battle over calories and putting a healthy lifestyle in place for good.

In addition to the eating plan attached to the Sardine Diet, you must drink at last two liters of water a day. The water serves several important purposes:

- Ω The neutral fluid takes the place of calorie-rich foods in filling you up and helping to prevent hunger, especially between meals.
- Ω Water helps flush your system, removing bad toxins and keeping your metabolism revved up.
- Ω It helps you avoid dehydration. Some symptoms of dehydration, such as lethargy and fatigue, mimic low blood sugar and might make you crave sweets or other high-calorie carbohydrates.

Saturday Night Splurge

If you're really serious about losing weight, you're going to have to give up dessert for a month or two. But come the weekend, everyone needs a treat. If you stick to the Sardine Diet all week, here's what you can allow yourself as a reward. Pick one:

Sweet Treats

1 ounce dark chocolate: sweet, semisweet, or bittersweet

15 frozen grapes

½ cup blueberries with ⅓ cup nonfat plain yogurt

2 high-fiber crackers with 2 teaspoons natural peanut butter

1 cup banana "ice cream": freeze chunks of peeled ripe banana, puree in a food processor or blender, then freeze again

3 large or 6 small strawberries with 1 tablespoon chocolate sauce

Maple-Walnut Baked Apple (recipe on page 89)

Grilled Pineapple Slices (recipe on page 89)

6 ounces nonfat plain yogurt mixed with 1 Swiss Miss® 20-calorie hot chocolate mix

You can also enjoy:

High-Fiber Fruits

Raspberries (1 cup): 8.6 g fiber

Pear with skin (1 medium): 4 g fiber

Blueberries (1 cup): 4 g fiber

Strawberries (1 cup): 3.8 g fiber

Fresh apricots (4): 3.4 g fiber

Fresh figs (2 medium): 3.3 g fiber

Peach (1 large): 3.1 g fiber

Apple (1 medium): 3 g fiber

Orange (1 medium): 3 g fiber

Mango (1 cup): 3 g fiber

Papaya (1 cup): 2.5 g fiber

Banana (1 medium) 2 g fiber

Pineapple (1 cup): 2 g fiber

Grapefruit (½ grapefruit): 1.7 g fiber

Cantaloupe (1 cup chunks): 1 g fiber

Plum (1): 1 g fiber

Grapes (15): 0.8 g fiber

Benefits of Exercise

30 MINUTES OF EXERCISE BURNS OFF THE FOLLOWING CALORIES PER MINUTE (DEPENDING ON WEIGHT):

EXERCISE	120 lb	140 lb	160 lb	180 lb
Basketball	7.5	8.8	10.0	11.3
Bowling	1.2	1.4	1.6	1.9
Cycling (10 mph)	5.5	6.4	7.3	8.2
Dancing (aerobic)	7.4	8.6	9.8	11.1
Dancing (social)	2.9	3.3	3.7	4.2
Golf (pull/carry clubs)	4.6	5.4	6.2	7.0
Golf (power cart)	2.1	2.5	2.8	3.2
Hiking	4.5	5.2	6.0	6.7
Jogging	9.3	10.8	12.4	13.9
Running (9-minute mile)	11.4	13.2	15.1	17.0
Sitting, quietly	1.2	1.3	1.5	1.7
Skating (ice and roller)	5.9	6.9	7.9	8.8
Skiing (cross-country)	7.5	8.8	10.0	11.3
Skiing (water and downhill)	5.7	6.6	7.6	8.5
Swimming (crawl, moderate pace)	7.8	9.0	10.3	11.6
Tennis	6.0	6.9	7.9	8.9
Walking (fast)	6.5	7.6	8.7	9.7
Weight Training	6.6	7.6	8.7	9.8
Yardwork	5.0	5.9	6.7	7.5

In addition to drinking enough water while you're dieting, it's advisable to get to bed as early as you can. Staying up late often brings on the munchies. When you're tired, you crave sugar.

And don't forget exercise. In addition to resetting your metabolic engine so that it purrs at a more efficient speed, every minute you spend exercising is an investment in losing weight. It also helps lower cholesterol and blood pressure, increases bone density, and reduces stress.

Getting started on an exercise program can be difficult, but you'll have much more success if you pick something you can do consistently. Even if you begin with just two or three 20- to 30-minute sessions per week, it's a start. Once you're hooked, you can increase the frequency.

Exercise also helps relieve stress, and cortisol, the hormone released by constant stress, causes an accumulation of fat around the midsection. That may be why even gentle exercise, like yoga, can prevent the pound-a-year weight gain that most people experience in middle age.

How much weight will you lose on the Sardine Diet? Everyone is different, but if you follow the plan faithfully for the full four weeks, you will definitely see and feel a big difference. Your energy level will be higher, and you'll have an increased sense of well-being. You will definitely look better.

At the end of that time, if you feel you still need to lose more weight, simply repeat the Sardine Diet for another month. It is so well-balanced and rich in protein, calcium, good fats, and all the nutrients you need that staying on it longer will only benefit you more.

Moving on to Maintenance

When you've lost the number of pounds you wish, it's time to move on to maintenance. This modified version of the Sardine Diet will ensure that your weight stays stable and while it continues to give you all the excellent nutrition you've been enjoying while on the diet.

Maintenance allows you to take all the lessons you've learned and build on them. Stick to the outlines of the detailed menus, substituting meats and vegetables you like, keeping in mind the same portion control and limited use of cooking fats. Be sure you continue to enjoy the benefits of omega-3s with sardines or another oily fish. Eat them alone or as part of a salad or other dish at least three times a week.

Each day, give yourself another serving of fruit whenever you feel like it as well as another high-fiber grain, starch, or legume (lentils and beans) for lunch or dinner. Enjoy sweets in moderation, and, if you wish, a glass of wine with supper—at most, two or three times a week. And save those treats for special occasions, not on the fly when you're feeling stressed.

Following are some foods to incorporate into your maintenance diet:

High-Fiber Grains and Starches

¼ cup cooked millet

¼ cup soaked bulgur

¼ cup cooked quinoa

⅓ cup cooked brown rice

1 whole-wheat wrap with at least 5 grams of fiber, such as La Tortilla™

4 high-fiber crackers with at least 5 grams of fiber, such as GG® Scandinavian bran crispbread

1 slice whole-grain bread with at least 3 grams of fiber

1 small or ½ large whole-wheat pita

1 whole-grain waffle with at least 3 grams of fiber

1 small baked potato or sweet potato

½ cup cooked whole-wheat pasta, such as Barilla®, which is fortified with omega-3s

1 Thomas'® light whole multi-grain English muffin

½ cup cooked butternut or acorn squash

½ cup corn kernels

½ cup peas

½ cup cooked chickpeas, beans, or lentils

On the Sardine Diet, you can eat as many healthful green vegetables as you like:

Green Vegetables High in Antioxidants and Fiber

Spinach	Romaine lettuce
Asparagus	Escarole
Broccoli	Bok choy
Kale	Mustard greens
Swiss chard	Dandelion greens
Brussels sprouts	Green beans
Arugula	Zucchini
Mesclun (baby field greens)	Green peppers
Collard greens	Turnip greens

The Issue of Safety

Why specifically sardines? Why not cod liver or other fish oil? Fish oil, either in liquid or capsule form, is a dicey alternative. Since it is so concentrated, it can be high in pollutants, and subject to questionable manufacturing standards. Plus, pharmaceutical-grade fish oil is expensive, and many people find the taste unpleasant and the oil very hard to digest.

And why not salmon, tuna, or other oily fish? Of course, you can enjoy these alternatives occasionally, but for a regular diet, Nordic brisling sardines are by far the safest choice. Because they are small and therefore low on the oceanic food chain, and because they swim in ice-cold fjords that are notably free of contaminants, they have the least chance of containing PCBs, mercury, and other heavy metals. Farm-raised salmon has recently tested high for PCBs, thought to come from their feed. Wild salmon, particularly from the Pacific Northwest, contains fewer contaminants than farmed or even wild Atlantic salmon. Big fish, like tuna caught in the Atlantic (particularly farther south), contain dangerously high levels of mercury and other pollutants. When eating tuna, choose chunk light, rather than solid white; chunk light comes from a type of tuna that is generally less contaminated.

Sardines' northern habitat also influences their omega-3 levels. These essential fatty acids break down in heat. But the clear, cold, northern waters that spawn Nordic brisling sardines produce fish with omega-3 fatty acids of the highest concentration as well as the purest quality—far superior to that of sardines caught in warmer waters to the south.

Concentration of Omega-3 in Sardines and Seafood

in grams per 3½-ounce serving:

Nordic brisling sardines	5.10
Chinook salmon	3.04
Atlantic mackerel	2.18
Pink salmon	1.87
Albacore tuna, canned light	1.69
Sablefish	1.39
Rainbow trout, U.S. farmed	1.08
Pacific oysters	.84
Striped bass	.64
Catfish	.61
Alaskan king crab	.46
Pacific halibut	.45
Shrimp	.39
Flounder, yellowtail	.30
Haddock	.16

Shopping for Sardines

While you may find fresh grilled sardines on the menu in Portugal, the term "sardine" is most widely and appropriately used for a variety of canned fish. In fact, a sardine is not one particular species of fish, but a general term that refers to some eleven different species of ocean fish—including herring, pilchard, sild, sprats, and brisling—that are processed and canned. This piece of trivia alone tells you that not all sardines are created equal. Some are smaller, some are larger, and they can be caught and produced to various standards around the globe. So beware: there is a world of difference in quality, taste, and consistency. Here's how to select the best sardines.

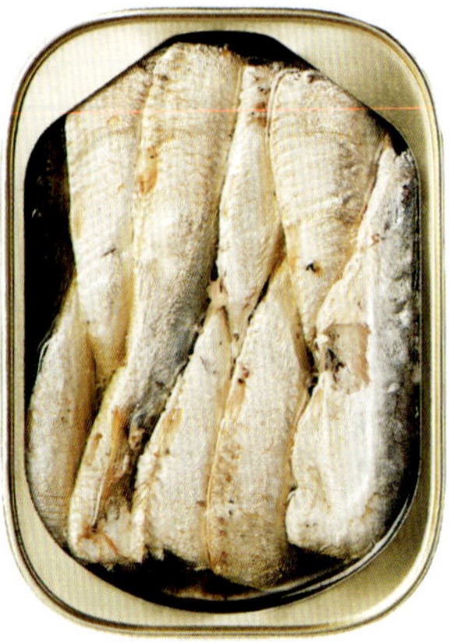

North Atlantic Sardines

Before you run out to the store to buy sardines, you need to know what to look for—you don't want to open the can only to find unappetizing bones or an unpleasant fishy smell. If this is what comes to mind when you think of sardines, you're not buying the right kind.

The best sardines are brisling sardines, specifically, Nordic brisling sardines. Brisling are tiny, tiny fish—among the very smallest used for sardines. This makes their bones imperceptible and their meat especially tender. Nordic brisling sardines are fished from clean, ice-cold waters using eco-friendly, sustainable methods. The cold environment elevates the omega-3 levels in the fish, and the purity of the water minimizes the risk of various pollutants and heavy metals such as mercury.

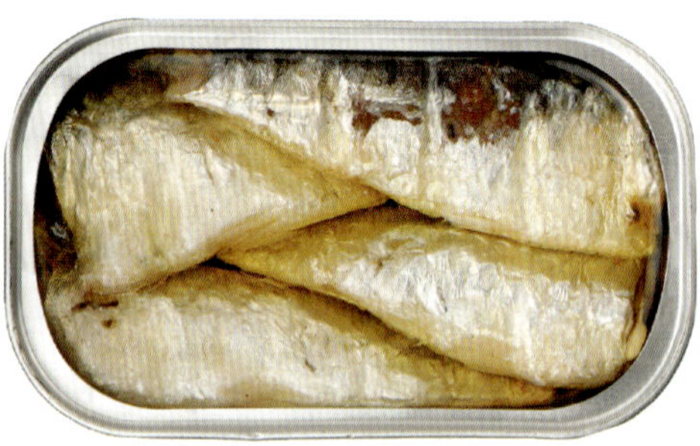

Portuguese Sardines

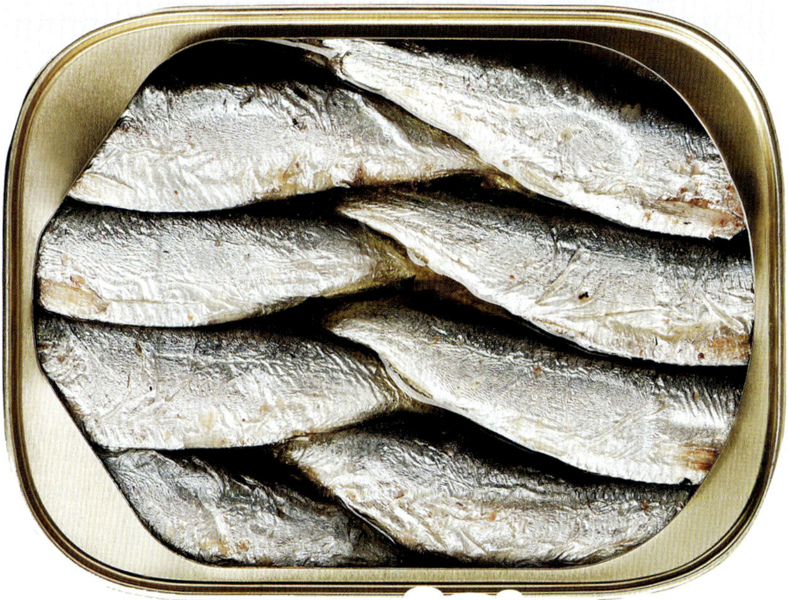

This can of brisling sardines comes from Norway. The fish are very small (as many as 24 in one 3.75-ounce can), and lightly smoked.

As a general rule, the smaller the sardine, the milder it is. There are noticeable differences between Nordic brisling and the North Sea herring used by most American and Canadian sardine manufacturers. These differences are even more pronounced when you look at the sardines commonly produced from various fish varieties caught in the waters off countries like Portugal, Thailand, or Morocco. The most obvious difference is size. Nordic brisling are uniformly smaller than the rest—just 3 to 4.5 inches long when fully mature. In contrast, the North Atlantic herring used for sardines by North American manufacturers average 8 to 10 inches in length. These larger fish are caught young, before the meat reaches peak quality, and then chopped up to fit into the can.

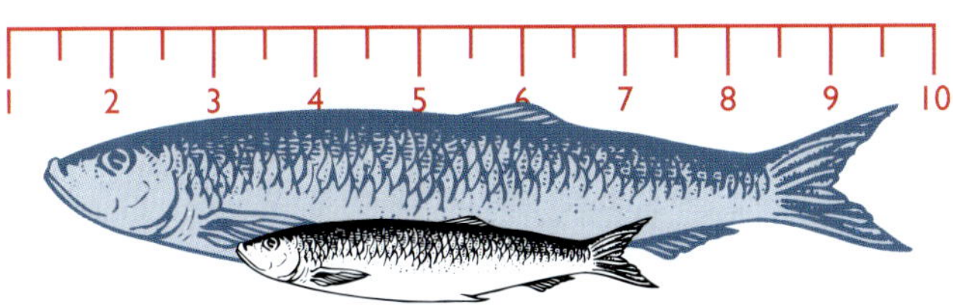

Chapter Four:

Health Benefits of the Sardine Diet

For decades, doctors and nutritionists have touted the advantages of one diet or another. Almost everyone has wrestled with their weight at one point in their lives. For the lucky ones, the extra pounds were brought on by a discrete event, such as the birth of a baby or giving up smoking. But for many, the struggle with the scale is an ongoing challenge. What's so special about the Sardine Diet is that it provides an eating plan that not only regulates weight but also visibly improves health in general. Here are some of the ways:

1. Weight loss and metabolic gains.
   Combined with exercise, the Sardine Diet's low-calorie menu plan provides an easy-to-follow path to guaranteed success in losing excess pounds and boosting metabolism.

2. Help avoid and control type 2 diabetes and "metabolic syndrome."
   Losing weight and reducing the amount of refined carbohydrates in your diet will help you avoid and control type 2 diabetes and "metabolic syndrome," which leads to diabetes. Maintaining blood sugar levels and avoiding sudden "peaks and valleys" is extremely beneficial to anyone who wants to feel and function their best. And it's critical to anyone suffering from any kind of diabetes.

3. Cardiovascular improvement.

The role of diet in cardiovascular health and high blood pressure has been well documented and is dramatic. The Sardine Diet can:

a) Raise "good" (HDL) and lower "bad" (LDL) cholesterol and triglyceride levels.

b) Lower blood pressure, especially important for people suffering from hypertension or those otherwise at risk for stroke.

c) Fight diseases of the arteries and the heart. The diet offers anticoagulant benefits, which keep the blood flowing and reduce the risk of strokes and heart attacks.

d) Omega-3s and a proper balance of fats help prevent both arteriosclerosis (hardening of the arteries) and atherosclerosis (buildup of plaque on the walls of the arteries).

e) Proper calcium and omega-3s help regulate heart rhythm.

4. Reduce suffering from anti-inflammatory and autoimmune diseases.

The right balance of fats, with plenty of omega-3 essential fatty acids and all the vitamins and minerals your body needs, can help reduce suffering from many autoimmune and anti-inflammatory diseases, such as arthritis, asthma, allergies, and psoriasis.

5. Reduce the risks of cancer.

The jury is still out on the complete relationship between omega-3 fatty acids and tumor development. There is much anecdotal evidence about fish oil and reduction of tumor size, but scientific studies have been inconclusive and, in some cases, disappointing. Many studies are still being followed.

What is known, though, is that omega-3s do help oxygenate tissues throughout the body, and they boost the immune system. Since your body is constantly working to spot, destroy, and remove cancerous cells—along with damaged cells, bad bacteria, and viruses—many doctors have concluded that there is a connection between omega-3s and better health, including their role in warding off certain types of cancer.

6. Encourage healthy pregnancies.

Calcium, from sardines and green leafy vegetables, is essential to the formation of bones in the developing fetus, as well as to replenishing that lost by the mother—both during pregnancy and while breastfeeding after birth. Folic acid from leafy greens is vital to babies' developing brains and neurological systems, especially in the first trimester. Omega-3s greatly facilitate cognitive development, including hearing and eyesight, particularly in the third trimester. Many studies suggest that they also help prevent miscarriage and premature birth. And since mercury is particularly damaging to the fetus, sardines are the best seafood choice during pregnancy. Finally, the high fiber of the Sardine Diet will be particularly welcome to pregnant women, because it gets the gastrointestinal (GI) tract moving and helps alleviate constipation.

7. Healthy skin.
   Both omega-3 fatty acids—with their anti-inflammatory and antioxidant properties—and antioxidants from vitamins A, C, and E help prevent the formation of wrinkles by keeping skin plump and hydrated. When all your tissues are well oxygenated, your color improves and your complexion becomes more youthful. Omega-3s also moisturize the skin from the inside out and give it better tone. Drinking enough water, which is an important part of the diet, will also help reduce the appearance of wrinkles.

8. Increase mental acuity and decrease depression.
   Your brain is largely made up of fat, and the spinal cord is sheathed with it. To function properly, your neurological system requires significant amounts of the kinds of omega-3s that you get only from sardines and other oily fish or seaweed. Mounting evidence suggests that the omega-3s may play a significant role in mood stabilization, helping to prevent depression and bipolar disorder. Proper amounts of dietary calcium have also been linked to reduced irritability and an increased sense of well-being.

Chapter Five: The Menu Plan & Recipes—A Month of Healthy Meals

FINALLY, what you've been waiting for: meals for a month that will help you lose weight and improve your health at the same time. At an average 1,250 calories a day, these meals are probably composed of less food than you are used to, but the bulk from all the high-fiber vegetables and grains should fill you up. Remember, whenever no amount is listed for a green vegetable you can eat all you want. If you're like most people, you'll start feeling a difference within just a few days. Your energy levels will rise, and your mood will improve. In all likelihood, you'll sleep better as well. Just don't forget the exercise.

Here are a few more tips to make sure the Sardine Diet works for you:

Snacks

Even though you're losing weight, on this plan you'll never be hungry, because you're allowed two snacks a day. You even get to choose your own snacks from the list. One is for midmorning and the other is eaten between lunch and dinner. Depending upon your personal schedule, this could be anywhere from 3 in the afternoon to 6 or even 7 in the evening, if you work late and don't eat dinner until 9 o'clock. The goal is to keep your blood sugar steady and to avoid those awful highs and lows that come from improper eating.

Each day, make one choice from the Vegetable Snacks and one from the Calcium Snacks (page 58). It's always best to vary your diet as much as possible, but you can eat whichever you prefer, as long as you stick with the routine.

About Beverages

You can have one cup of coffee or tea with caffeine in the morning. You are even allowed up to 1/4 cup skim milk or soy milk. After that, though, move on to decaf green tea (high in antioxidants), or herb teas.

In between meals, be sure to drink at least two liters (that's almost two quarts) of water. This fills you up, keeps you hydrated, and helps flush out toxins.

Begin each day with a glass of warm water and a lemon wedge. (That's for squeezing into the glass, *not* decoration.) This mildly tart drink, taken first thing in the morning, provides several benefits:

- It's refreshing, and it helps you start the day with a healthy mind-set. Much of the success of dieting is your attitude and commitment, and being in the right frame of mind first thing can help with both of those.

- Fresh lemon both detoxifies the liver and delivers a nice dose of vitamin C. (That orange juice you're used to drinking is much too high in sugar and calories.)

- The warm drink (which is actually alkaline in nature, even though the lemon tastes acidic) helps get your GI tract moving. The earlier you eliminate, the better.

Preparing the Food

Some of the meals in the weekly plans contain little mini-recipes within them. Others refer you to some of the excellent sardine recipes at the back of the book, occasionally with minor changes to accommodate the initial stages of the diet, which require greater calorie reduction. After you reach maintenance, feel free to enjoy any of the sardine recipes as many times a week as you like.

Wherever a meat or a fish is listed and there are no directions, you may cook it any way you like. You can bake, broil, grill, or sauté, as long as you use only a light mist of nonstick vegetable spray. Keep in mind, though, that because the omega-3s are susceptible to heat, light steaming is the cooking method of choice for fish as well as for green vegetables.

Sweets

No dessert? No surprise there. If you really want to lose weight, cutting out sugar and refined carbohydrates is a must. Given that the Sardine Diet includes all the major food groups, some satisfyingly sweet fruits are prescribed, especially those high in fiber, but these are included in breakfasts and lunches. Like a smoker quitting smoking, it's best to wean yourself of bad habits, such as always having something sweet after dinner. This is one sacrifice you're going to have to make. But once a week, you can reward yourself with a Sweet Treat from the list on page 33.

Go for It!

Okay, now you're armed with all the information you need about Nordic brisling sardines and your health. You've got the diet plans and the recipes. The rest is up to you. Four weeks and you'll be sold for a lifetime. Give the Sardine Diet a chance to work for you and you'll be hooked!

Sunday	Monday	Tuesday
Oatmeal Pancake (page 90) Warm water with lemon Coffee or tea	1 slice whole-wheat toast 1 hard-boiled egg ½ grapefruit Warm water with lemon Coffee or tea	Oatmeal with Almonds ½ cup oatmeal flakes ½ cup skim milk 8 almonds Sprinkle with cinnamon Warm water with lemon Coffee or tea
Chopped Salad with Toasted Sardines and Walnuts (page 65)	Chef's Salad 2 cups romaine lettuce 2 ounces lean ham or roast beef 2 ounces turkey ½ cup cherry tomatoes ½ cup diced cucumbers 1 ounce reduced-fat Cheddar cheese, diced 1-inch slice avocado, cut into chunks Splash of balsamic or red wine vinegar	Tofu Salad 1 cup shelled edamame ¼ cup diced firm tofu ¼ cup thinly sliced red and yellow bell peppers ¼ cup chopped celery ¼ cup chopped carrot 1 teaspoon sesame oil Rice vinegar to taste
Turkey Burger 4 ounces ground turkey breast, seasoned to taste and grilled or broiled Steamed kale 1 small baked sweet potato Mixed green salad 2 tablespoons *Vinaigrette (page 87)*	*Keri's Broiled Chicken (page 88)* 6 ounces broiled chicken breast on the bone, skin removed Steamed broccoli Mixed cherry tomato and chopped greens 2 tablespoons *Vinaigrette (page 87)*	*Spinach Salad with Grilled Tofu and Sardines (page 64* (omit sugar)

Wednesday	Thursday	Friday	Saturday
ambled Egg with oked Salmon ge 91) ice light whole-wheat ad, toasted rm water with lemon fee or tea	*Breakfast Burrito (page 92)* Warm water with lemon Coffee or tea	2 slices turkey bacon 1 slice wheat toast 1 cup mango chunks Warm water with lemon Coffee or tea	Cold Cereal with Walnuts ½ cup cold cereal 1 cup skim milk 1 tablespoon chopped walnuts Warm water with lemon Coffee or tea
lnut-Goat Cheese Salad cups mesclun greens ounce crumbled goat cheese tablespoons chopped walnuts chopped figs teaspoon extra virgin olive oil alsamic vinegar or wine vinegar to taste	Steak Salad 2 cups baby spinach 3 ounces grilled lean steak, thinly sliced ½ cup cherry tomatoes 2 tablespoons chopped red onion 1 teaspoon *Vinaigrette (page 87)*	*Two-Cheese Caesar Salad (page 66)* (omit croutons)	Cobb Salad 2 cups shredded romaine lettuce 2 ounces turkey bacon, cooked and crumbled ¼ cup cherry tomatoes ½ cup diced cucumbers 1 hard-boiled egg white, finely diced 1-inch slice avocado, cut into chunks 1 teaspoon olive oil Splash of vinegar
key Cutlet -ounce turkey cutlet, seasoned to taste and grilled or broiled amed spinach with on juice ed green salad blespoon vinaigrette	Tofu Kebab 4 ounces tofu cubes skewered with mushrooms and squares of red and yellow bell pepper and onion, grilled or broiled Broiled bok choy ¼ cup quinoa, rinsed and cooked Mixed green salad 2 tablespoons *Vinaigrette (page 87)*	Tilapia 4-ounce fresh tilapia fillet, seasoned to taste and grilled or broiled Steamed broccoli Mixed green salad 1 tablespoon *Vinaigrette (page 87)*	Hamburger 4 ounces lean ground beef, seasoned to taste Steamed spinach with lemon juice Mixed green salad 2 tablespoons *Vinaigrette (page 87)*

Sunday	Monday	Tuesday
Omega Spread (page 84) 4 tablespoons spread on 4 fiber crackers 1 cup blueberries Warm water with lemon Coffee or tea	*Breakfast Burrito (page 92)* Warm water with lemon Coffee or tea	Cold Cereal with Walnuts Warm water with lemon Coffee or tea
Roasted Chicken Lettuce Wraps (page 87)	Vegetable Cottage Cheese Salad ½ cup 1% fat cottage cheese ⅓ cup chopped vegetables (onion or scallion, celery, carrots or peppers and tomatoes and cucumber) 2 cups chopped romaine lettuce 1 tablespoon *Vinaigrette (page 87)*	Vegetable "Sushi" 2 Vegetable handrolls with avocado, no rice 1 cup edamame 1 cup miso soup
Scallops 4 ounces scallops, seasoned to taste and grilled Steamed asparagus Mixed green salad 2 tablespoons *Vinaigrette (page 87)*	Hamburger 4 ounces lean ground beef, seasoned to taste and grilled or broiled 1 small whole wheat pita Steamed spinach with lemon Mixed green salad 2 tablespoons *Vinaigrette (page 87)*	Chicken Paillard 4-ounce grilled chicken cutlet with a squeeze of lemon juice Steamed Brussels sprouts ½ cup whole wheat pasta with ¼ cup marinara sauce Mixed green salad 2 tablespoons *Vinaigrette (page 87)*

Wednesday	Thursday	Friday	Saturday
eddar-Broccoli Omelet ge 91) rm water with lemon fee or tea	*Yogurt Parfait (page 93)* Warm water with lemon Coffee or tea	Smoked Salmon and Toast 1 slice whole wheat toast 2 ounces smoked salmon 1 slice tomato 1 thin slice onion Squeeze of lemon juice ½ grapefruit Warm water with lemon Skim latte or tea	*French Toast (page 92)* Warm water with lemon Coffee or tea
lnut-Goat Cheese Salad	Steak Salad	*Spinach Omelet with Tomatoes and Parmesan Cheese (page 90)*	*Fennel Salad with Sardines, Clementines, and Pickled Onions (page 68)*
k Tenderloin ounces pork tenderloin, seasoned to taste and roasted or grilled amed green beans ed green salad blespoons *Vinaigrette ge 87)*	*Linguini with Fresh Fennel and Sardines (page 77)* Mixed green salad 2 tablespoons *Vinaigrette (page 87)*	Tofu Kebab Broiled bok choy Mixed green salad 2 tablespoons *Vinaigrette (page 87)*	*Keri's Broiled Chicken (page 88)* 4 ounces broiled chicken Steamed broccoli Mixed green salad 2 tablespoons *Vinaigrette (page 87)*

Sunday	Monday	Tuesday
1 slice whole-wheat bread, toasted 1 hard-boiled egg 1 cup sliced strawberries Warm water with lemon Coffee or tea	Oatmeal with Almonds Warm water with lemon Coffee or tea	Cold Cereal with Walnuts Warm water with lemon Coffee or tea
Roasted Chicken Lettuce Wraps (page 87)	*Asian Slaw with Sardines, Scallions and Sesame Seeds (page 72)*	Chef's Salad
Pork Tenderloin 4 ounces pork tenderloin, seasoned to taste and roasted or grilled Roasted green beans Mixed green salad 2 tablespoons *Vinaigrette (page 87)*	*Keri's Broiled Chicken (page 88)* 4 ounces broiled chicken Steamed escarole $\frac{1}{3}$ cup wild rice Mixed green salad 2 tablespoons *Vinaigrette (page 87)*	Steamed Shrimp 4 ounces steamed medium shrimp Steamed asparagus Mixed green salad 2 tablespoons *Vinaigrette (page 87)* 1 cup mango chunks

Wednesday	Thursday	Friday	Saturday
nch Toast (page 92) rm water with lemon fee or tea	*Yogurt Parfait (page 93)* Warm water with lemon Coffee or tea	*Cheddar-Broccoli Omelet (page 91)* 2 to 4 high-fiber crackers Warm water with lemon Coffee or tea	*Pita Pockets with Lemony Hummus, Sardines, and Olives (page 82)* Warm water with lemon Skim latte or tea
etable "Sushi" egetable hand-rolls h avocado (no rice) up edamame up miso soup range	Tofu Salad	Bean Salad 1 cup mixed beans (any combination of cannelini, pinto beans, black beans, kidney beans, or chickpeas) 1 tablespoon chopped onion 1 teaspoon lime juice Salt and pepper 2 cups chopped romaine lettuce 1 tablespoon *Vinaigrette (page 87)*	Vegetable Cottage Cheese Salad
key Cutlet ounces turkey cutlet, seasoned to taste and grilled or broiled amed spinach ed green salad blespoons *Vinaigrette* *ge 87)*	*Sardine Pasta Primavera (page 72)* ½ cup pasta Mixed green salad 2 tablespoons *Vinaigrette (page 87)*	Tilapia 4 ounces tilapia fillet, seasoned to taste and broiled or grilled Steamed broccoli 1 small sweet potato Mixed green salad 2 tablespoons *Vinaigrette (page 87)*	Fillet of Beef 4 ounces beef tenderloin, seasoned to taste and roasted or grilled Steamed asparagus Mixed green salad 2 tablespoons *Vinaigrette (page 87)*

Sunday	Monday	Tuesday
Breakfast Burrito (page 92) Warm water with lemon Coffee or tea	*Deviled Sardine Spread (page 84)* 4 tablespoons spread on 4 high-fiber crackers Warm water with lemon Coffee or tea	*French Toast (page 92)* Warm water with lemon Coffee or tea
Cobb Salad 1 orange	*Spinach Omelet with Tomatoes and Parmesan Cheese (page 90)*	Walnut-Goat Cheese Salad
Scallops 4 ounces scallops, seasoned to taste and grilled Grilled bok choy Grilled Portobello mushroom Mixed green salad 2 tablespoons *Vinaigrette (page 87)*	Chicken Paillard 4 ounces grilled chicken cutlet with a squeeze of lemon juice Steamed Brussels sprouts Mixed green salad 2 tablespoons *Vinaigrette (page 87)*	Shrimp Marinara 4 ounces peeled shrimp ¼ cup jarred marinara sauce ½ cup whole-wheat pasta Steamed escarole Mixed green salad 2 tablespoons *Vinaigrette (page 87)*

Wednesday	Thursday	Friday	Saturday
ddar-Broccoli Omelet *ge 91)* rm water with lemon fee or tea	*Oatmeal Pancake* *(page 90)* Warm water with lemon Coffee or tea	*Yogurt Parfait* *(page 93)* Warm water with lemon Coffee or tea	Cold Cereal with Walnuts Warm water with lemon Coffee or tea
hard Fresh Sardine *ad (page 74)* (omit atoes)	Tofu Salad	*Roasted Chicken Lettuce* *Wraps (page 87)*	Chef Salad
diterranean Plate 2 tablespoons *Lemony Hummus* *(page 83)* Cut up raw vegetables: carrots, cucumbers, bell peppers, celery, radishes 5 olives 1 veggie burger xed green salad blespoons *Vinaigrette* *ge 87)*	Turkey Burger 4 ounces ground turkey breast, seasoned to taste and grilled or broiled Steamed kale 1 small baked sweet potato Mixed green salad 2 tablespoons *Vinaigrette* *(page 87)*	*Whole-Wheat Pita Pizzas* *with Anchovies, Browned* *Onion, and Sweet Red* *Pepper (page 81)*	*Keri's Broiled Chicken* *(page 88)* 4 ounces broiled chicken Steamed broccoli Mixed green salad 2 tablespoons *Vinaigrette* *(page 87)*

Vegetable Snacks

Celery sticks sprinkled with kosher salt and/or 1 tablespoon ground flaxseeds

1 cup sliced red and yellow bell peppers dipped in 1 tablespoon salsa

1 cup *Carrot-Cabbage Slaw (page 86)* in a seaweed wrap

1 cup sugar snap peas

1 cup sliced cucumbers sprinkled with rice vinegar

1 cup cherry tomatoes

1 cup chopped cucumbers and carrots sprinkled with fresh lemon juice and 1 tablespoon ground flaxseeds

Calcium Snacks

1 (6- to 8-ounce) nonfat plain yogurt with 1 tablespoon ground flaxseeds and 2 high-fiber crackers
Variation: Same as above, with yogurt frozen

½ cup 1% cottage cheese with cinnamon and 1 tablespoon ground flaxseeds with 2 high-fiber crackers

1 skim decaf latte with 2 high-fiber crackers

1 low sugar nonfat yogurt shake with 2 high-fiber crackers

1 tablespoon *Savory Spinach Dip (page 86)* with 2 high-fiber crackers and sliced cucumbers

1 ounce low-fat cheese with 2 high-fiber crackers

2 tablespoons *Omega Spread (page 84)* with 2 high-fiber crackers

12 almonds or 1 tablespoon almond butter on 2 high-fiber crackers

2 *Cucumber-Sardine Tea Sandwiches (page 80)*

2 tablespoons *Sardine Pâté (page 105),* made with nonfat mayonnaise, on 2 high-fiber crackers

Keri's Picks

Brands vary across the country, but here are a few of my favorite healthy foods:

SARDINES King Oscar® is the brand that ensures you're getting Nordic brisling sardines from cold, clear waters for the highest omega-3 count.

HIGH-FIBER CRACKERS Look for crackers with a minimum of 5 grams of fiber, preferably higher. My favorites are FiberRich® and GG® Scandinavian Bran CrispBread.

HIGH-FIBER TORTILLAS Look for La Tortilla™ whole-wheat tortillas.

VEGGIE BURGERS Dr. Praeger's® and Gardenburger® are good brands that can be found in health food stores as well as in the health food sections of many supermarkets.

The Recipes

ABOUT THIS CHAPTER:
The first section contains the recipes best suited to the weight-loss menu plan. Once you have met your weight-loss goals, you can enjoy the recipes in the second section, which are also rich in omega-3.

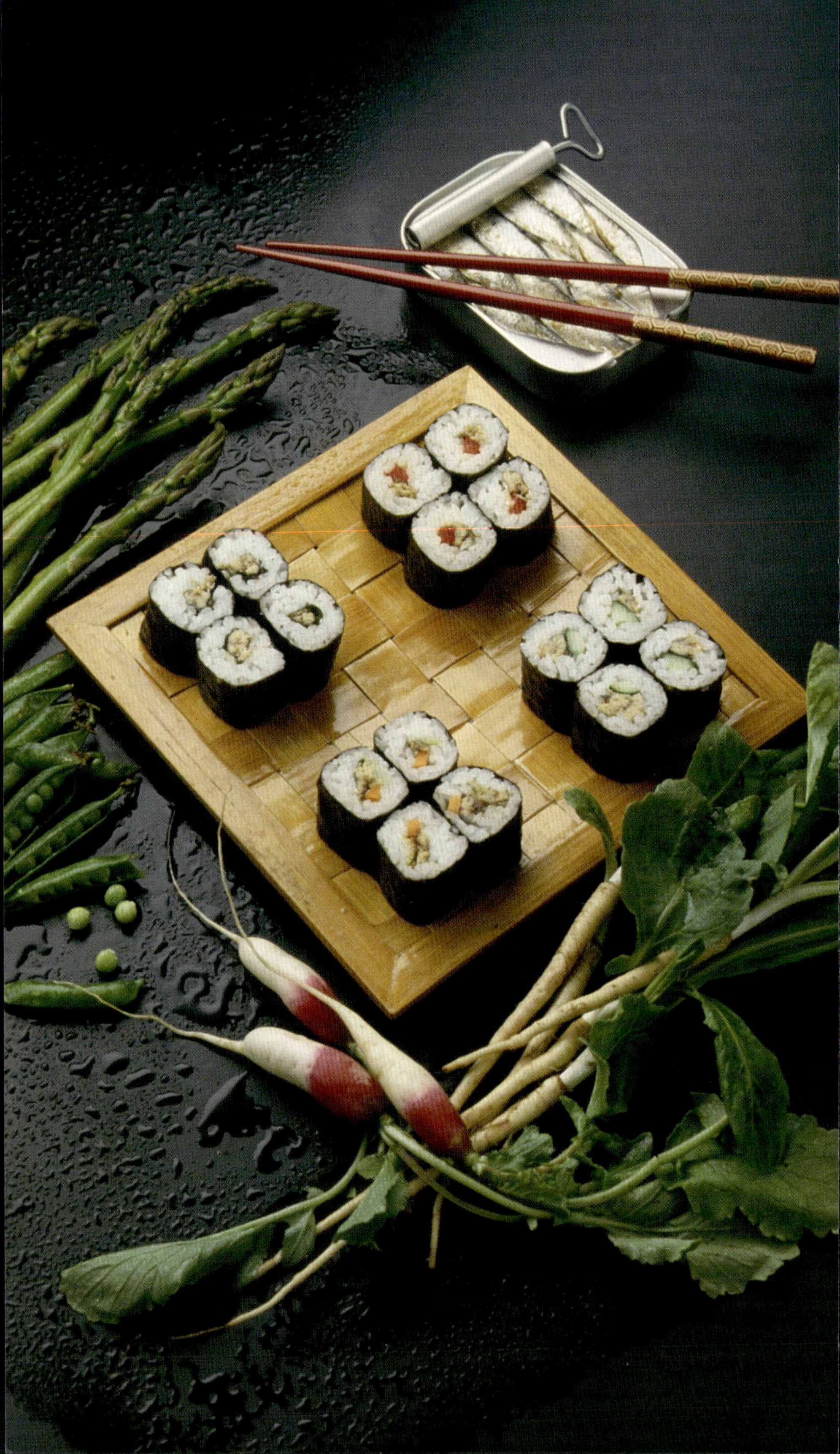

Sardine Sushi

MAKES ABOUT 30 PIECES

2 cups short-grain brown rice, rinsed

2 teaspoons sugar

3 tablespoons unseasoned rice vinegar

4 sheets nori (dried seaweed), about 6x8 inches each

2 cans (3.75 ounces each) Nordic brisling sardines in olive oil, drained

Vegetables cut into thin julienne (carrots, scallions, cucumbers, radishes)

1. Cook the rice in a large saucepan with 2 ¾ cups water, covered, until the water is absorbed, about 40 minutes. Remove rice from heat and let stand, still covered, for 10 minutes longer. Spread out rice on a baking sheet. In a small bowl, stir sugar into vinegar until it dissolves; sprinkle over rice and toss to mix. Let rice cool completely.
2. To assemble the sushi, place a piece of nori, shiny side down, on a bamboo sushi mat with a long side facing you. Spread about one-fourth of the seasoned rice evenly over the nori, leaving a 1-inch margin at top edge. Arrange sardines across center of rice. Top with an even layer of vegetables. Starting from bottom, use mat to roll up the nori, enclosing the filling. Press the mat gently around the roll to shape it, then moisten the top edge of the nori with water and seal the roll snugly.
3. Remove the mat; press in loose ends. Place the sushi roll seam-side down on cutting board. Repeat with the remaining nori and filling. Slice the roll into 1-inch rounds with a large sharp knife, dipped in water, and wiped dry between each cut.

Spinach Salad with Grilled Tofu and Sardines

Serves 2 or 3

High in lean protein and rich in omega-3s, this is the perfect Sardine Diet salad. Best of all, it can be thrown together in little more time than it takes to open a can. Garnish, if you like, with cherry tomatoes.

1 cake extra-firm tofu, seasoned to taste

1 package (10 ounces) washed baby spinach

½ white onion, thinly sliced

1 tablespoon extra-virgin olive oil

1 tablespoon sesame oil

1 tablespoon rice-wine vinegar

1 teaspoon soy sauce

¼ teaspoon sugar

Salt and freshly ground black pepper

2 cans (3.75 ounces each) Nordic brisling sardines, drained

1. Heat a nonstick ridged stove-top grill pan over medium-high heat until hot. Add the tofu and cook for 2 to 3 minutes, until grill marks appear; rotate 90 degrees. Grill until a crosshatch pattern appears, 2 to 3 minutes longer. Turn the tofu over with a spatula and repeat on the second side. Transfer to a plate and let cool slightly. Cut the tofu into cubes.

2. Place the spinach and onion slices in a large bowl. Sprinkle with the olive oil, sesame oil, vinegar, soy sauce, and sugar; toss to mix. Season with salt and pepper to taste. Add the tofu cubes and toss again.

3. Divide the salad among 2 or 3 plates. Arrange the sardines on top.

Chopped Salad with Sardines and Toasted Walnuts

Makes 4 to 6 servings

⅓ cup walnuts

1 small head of romaine or iceberg lettuce

2 ribs celery, diced

2 carrots, peeled and diced

1 cup diced seedless cucumber

1 cup broccoli or cauliflower florets (lightly steamed, if desired), diced

1 cup diced roasted or pickled beets

¾ cup diced red or green bell pepper

½ cup finely diced white onion

3 tablespoons chopped fresh parsley

3 tablespoons extra-virgin olive oil

1 tablespoon walnut oil (or use an extra tablespoon olive oil)

2½ tablespoons sherry, balsamic, or red-wine vinegar

1 teaspoon dried oregano

Salt and freshly ground black pepper

2 cans (3.75 ounces each) Nordic brisling sardines, drained

1. Heat the oven to 325°F. Spread the walnuts in a baking dish and toast until fragrant, 6 to 8 minutes. Transfer to a plate and let cool, then coarsely chop.
2. Chop enough lettuce to measure 4 cups; put it in a large salad bowl. Add the celery, carrots, cucumber, broccoli, beets, bell pepper, onion, and half of the parsley and walnuts. Toss to mix.
3. In a small bowl, whisk together the olive oil, walnut oil, vinegar, and oregano. Season with salt and pepper to taste. Pour over the salad and toss well to coat evenly.
4. Divide the salad among 4 pasta bowls or plates. Arrange the sardines on top. Garnish with the remaining parsley and walnuts.

Two-Cheese Caesar Salad

Serves 4 to 6

Tangy blue cheese combined with Parmesan makes for a Caesar salad sure to bring raves from your guests.

1 large head romaine lettuce or 2 romaine hearts

2 slices multigrain or high-fiber bread

Vegetable cooking spray, preferably olive oil

1 clove garlic, crushed through a press

1 teaspoon Worcestershire sauce

1 can (3.75 ounces) Nordic brisling sardines in oil, drained

3 tablespoons fresh lemon juice

¼ cup olive oil

Freshly ground black pepper

1½ ounces blue cheese, such as Maytag Blue, Roquefort, or Bleu d'Auvergne, crumbled (about 3 tablespoons)

3 tablespoons freshly grated Parmesan cheese

1. Heat the oven to 375°F. Tear the lettuce into large bite-size pieces or cut crosswise into ½-inch slices. Rinse in a large bowl of cold water and spin dry. Place in a plastic bag and chill until ready to toss.
2. Cut the bread into ½-inch cubes. Place on a baking sheet and coat lightly with the vegetable spray. Toss and spray again. Bake for 5 minutes; toss. Continue to bake until the croutons are crisp and lightly toasted, 5 to 7 minutes longer.
3. In a large salad bowl, combine the garlic and Worcestershire sauce. Add half the sardines and coarsely mash with a fork, leaving little pieces intact. Stir in the lemon juice, olive oil, and pepper to taste.
4. Add the lettuce to the dressing in the bowl and toss to coat. Sprinkle with half the blue cheese and Parmesan and toss to mix. Top the salad with the remaining cheese and sardines and serve.

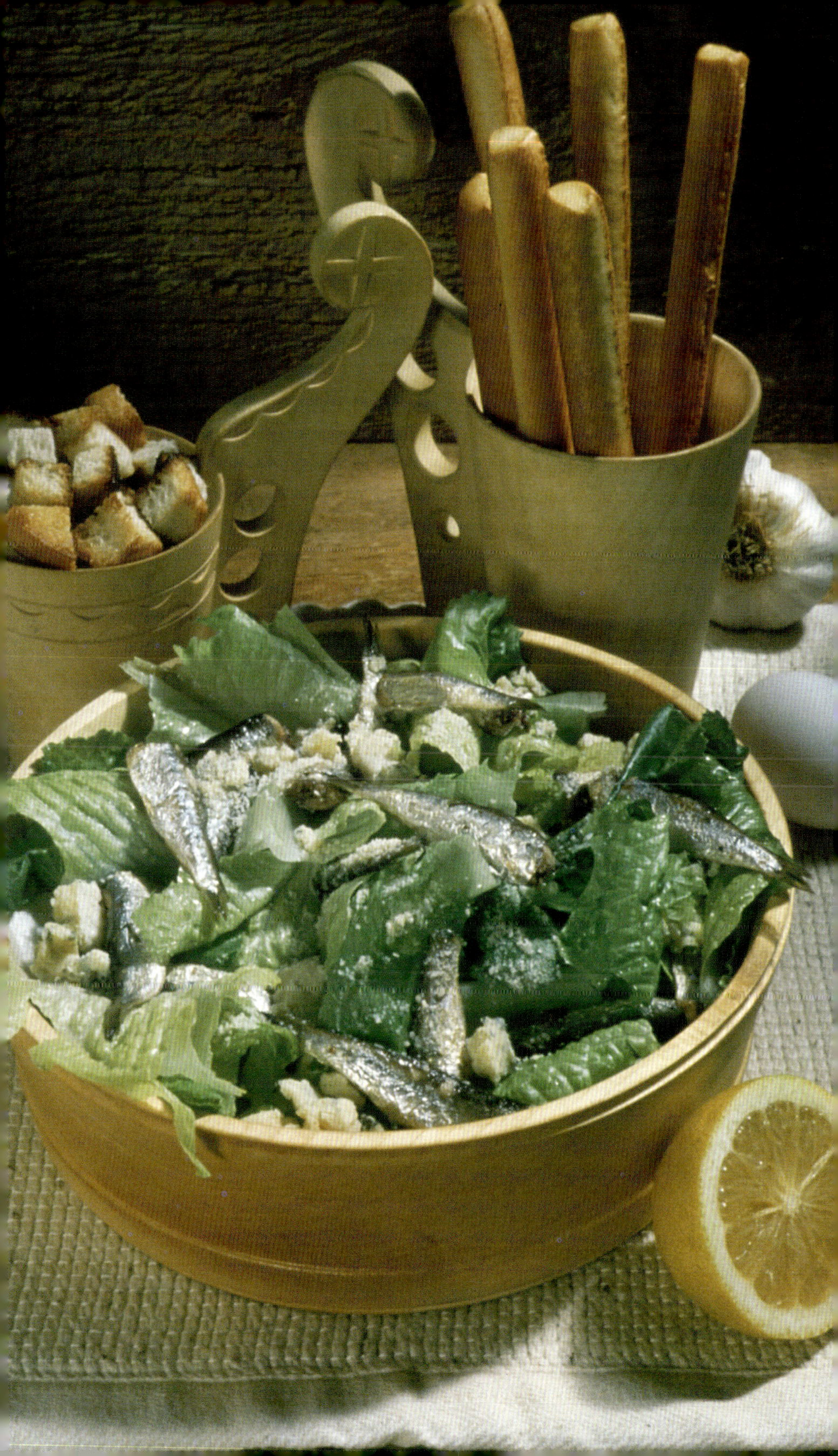

Fennel Salad with Sardines, Clementines, and Pickled Onio

MAKES 4 TO 6 SERVINGS

Orange segments are traditional in this recipe (and you can substitute them if you prefer), but clementines are charming and involve less work.

1 medium red onion, sliced into paper-thin rings

2 tablespoons orange juice

1½ tablespoons sherry vinegar

1 tablespoon balsamic vinegar

½ teaspoon coarse salt

3 tablespoons extra-virgin olive oil

2 bulbs fresh fennel

4 cups salad greens of your choice (mesclun, arugula, mache, frisée, torn romaine)

3 or 4 clementines, peeled and divided into sections

2 cans (3.75 ounces each) Nordic brisling sardines, drained

Coarsely ground black pepper

1. Place the red onion in a small bowl or container. Add the orange juice, sherry vinegar, balsamic vinegar, and salt. Cover and marinate for at least 2 hours at room temperature or overnight in the refrigerator.
2. Drain the onion slices, reserving the juices. Whisk the olive oil into the juices to make a vinaigrette.
3. Using a mandoline or food processor, slice the fennel paper-thin. On a large platter or shallow serving dish, make a bed of the greens. Place the fennel on top of the lettuce and drizzle on the vinaigrette.
4. Scatter the clementine sections over the fennel. Arrange the sardines on top and garnish with the pickled onion slices. Sprinkle the salad with a pinch of coarse black pepper.

Potato and Apple Salad with Sardines

MAKES 4 SERVINGS

¾ pound small red potatoes, cooked, drained, and sliced ¼-inch thick

2 small red apples, cored and thinly sliced

¼ cup extra-virgin olive oil

1½ tablespoons lemon juice

1 teaspoon Dijon mustard

1 teaspoon mustard seeds

1½ teaspoons chopped fresh dill or ½ teaspoon dried dill weed

½ teaspoon grated lemon zest

2 scallions, thinly sliced

Freshly ground black pepper

2 cans (3.75 ounces each) Nordic brisling sardines in oil, drained

Lettuce leaves, sprigs of fresh dill, and lemon wedges, for garnish

1. In a large bowl, combine the potato and apple slices. In a small bowl, whisk together the olive oil, lemon juice, mustard, mustard seeds, dill, lemon zest, scallions, and pepper. Pour the dressing over the potato and apple slices; toss to coat. Cover and refrigerate until chilled.
2. To serve, line each plate with lettuce leaves. Arrange the potato and apple salad and the sardines on top, dividing equally. Garnish with dill sprigs and lemon wedges.

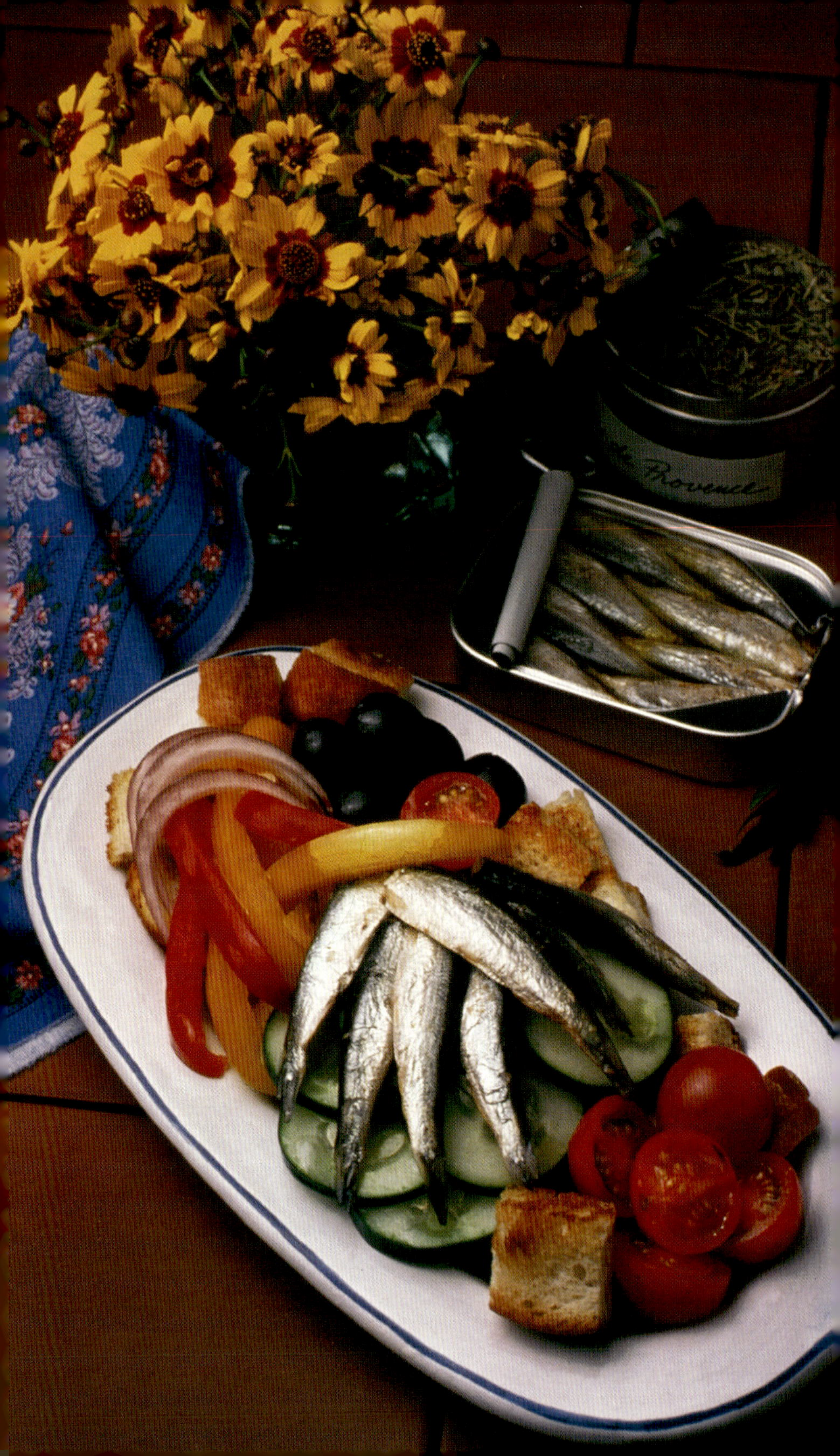
Provence

Sardine Salad Provençal

Makes 4 servings

Provençal Dressing (recipe follows)

1 cup halved cherry tomatoes

1 cup sliced cucumbers

1 small red onion, thinly sliced

1 red, yellow, or green bell pepper, cut into strips

½ cup pitted kalamata or niçoise olives

2 cups whole grain bread cubes (1-inch), toasted in oven

2 cans (3.75 ounces each) Nordic brisling sardines in oil, drained

1. Prepare the dressing as described below. Add tomatoes, cucumbers, onion, bell pepper, and olives to dressing; toss.
2. Line a serving dish or deep platter with the toast cubes. Top with the vegetables and sardines. Pour any remaining dressing over the salad. Serve immediately.

Provençal Dressing

1 clove garlic, slightly crushed

⅓ cup extra-virgin olive oil

3 tablespoons red-wine vinegar

½ teaspoon fresh thyme leaves

½ teaspoon chopped fresh tarragon

Salt and freshly ground black pepper

Rub a large bowl with the garlic clove. Add olive oil, vinegar, and herbs; whisk to blend. Season to taste with salt and pepper. Remove garlic before using dressing.

Asian Slaw with Sardines, Scallions, and Sesame Seed

Makes 4 servings

6 cups shredded green cabbage

3 medium carrots, peeled and coarsely shredded

1 medium red bell pepper (or use ½ green and ½ red), cut into very thin slices 1 to 1½ inches long

2 cans (3.75 ounces each) Nordic brisling sardines, drained

⅓ cup Sesame-Ginger Vinaigrette (recipe follows)

1½ tablespoons toasted sesame seeds

3 tablespoons thinly sliced scallions

1. In a salad bowl, combine the cabbage, carrots, and bell pepper. Toss to mix.
2. Drizzle the Sesame-Ginger Vinaigrette over the vegetables and toss. Let stand for 5 to 10 minutes to allow the dressing to soak into the vegetables.
3. Mound the slaw on a platter or divide among 4 plates. Dust with the sesame seeds. Arrange the sardines over the slaw and sprinkle the scallions on top.

Sesame-Ginger Vinaigrette

Makes about ⅓ cup

3 tablespoons extra-virgin olive oil

3 tablespoons rice-wine vinegar

2 teaspoons Asian sesame oil

1 teaspoon soy sauce

1 teaspoon minced fresh ginger

Place all the ingredients in a jar. Add 2 tablespoons water, close the lid tightly, and shake.

Tricolor Sardine Salad

MAKES 4 SERVINGS

6 Boston or red leaf lettuce leaves, washed and dried

2 cans (3.75 ounces each) Nordic brisling sardines in oil, drained

1 bunch fresh beets, cooked, drained, peeled and sliced, or 1 can (16 ounces) sliced beets, drained

1 medium cucumber, sliced

⅓ cup thinly sliced white onion

Lemon wedges, for garnish

Green Horseradish Dressing (recipe follows)

Line a shallow bowl with the lettuce leaves. Arrange the sardines and beet and cucumber slices decoratively over the lettuce. Scatter sliced onion on top. Garnish with lemon wedges. Serve Green Horseradish Dressing on the side.

Green Horseradish Dressing

MAKES ABOUT ⅓ CUP

2 tablespoons extra-virgin olive oil

2 tablespoons lemon juice

2 tablespoons water

4 teaspoons prepared white horseradish

1 teaspoon sugar

⅓ cup sliced scallions

Salt

In a mini food processor or blender, combine the oil, lemon juice, water, horseradish, sugar, and scallions. Puree until smooth. Season with salt to taste.

Orchard-Fresh Sardine Salad

MAKES 4 SERVINGS

2 cups fresh spinach leaves, washed and chilled

½ pound small red potatoes, cooked, drained, and quartered

2 cans (3.75 ounces each) Nordic brisling sardines in oil, drained

1 large tart green apple (such as Granny Smith), cored and cut into thin slices

1 small red onion, sliced and separated into rings

2 tablespoons chopped parsley

Apple-Orange Dressing (recipe follows)

Line a large platter with the spinach. Arrange the potatoes, sardines, apples, and onion on top. Garnish with parsley. Serve the Apple-Orange Dressing on the side.

Apple-Orange Dressing

MAKES ABOUT ⅔ CUP

¼ cup unsweetened apple juice

¼ cup extra-virgin olive oil

2 tablespoons apple-cider vinegar

½ teaspoon dry mustard

½ teaspoon grated orange zest

Salt

In a small bowl, whisk together the apple juice, vinegar, mustard, and orange zest. Whisk in the olive oil and season with salt to taste.

Frisée and Sardine Salad

Makes 2 servings

- 1 head frisée lettuce
- 1 bunch watercress
- 3 to 4 tablespoons raspberry vinegar
- ¼ cup extra-virgin olive oil
- 1 clove garlic
- 1 teaspoon Dijon mustard
- 8 to 12 small cherry tomatoes, halved
- 4 hard-boiled eggs, quartered
- 1 or 2 cans (3.75 ounces each) Nordic brisling sardines, drained

1. Rinse and dry the frisée and watercress. Tear into small pieces and put in a salad bowl.
2. In a small bowl, whisk together the vinegar, olive oil, garlic, and mustard. Pour the dressing over the salad and toss well. Divide the salad between 2 plates. Top with the tomatoes, eggs, and sardines, and serve right away.

Warm Winter Salad

Makes 4 servings

Warm Dill Dressing (recipe follows)

Florets from 1 bunch broccoli

2 large carrots, peeled and thickly sliced on the diagonal

2 medium leeks (white and tender green parts only), well rinsed

2 cups shredded red cabbage

2 cans (3.75 ounces each) Nordic brisling sardines in oil, drained

Dill sprigs, for garnish

1. Make Warm Dill Dressing; set aside. Briefly steam the broccoli, carrots, and leeks, separately, just until crisp-tender; drain immediately. Cut the leeks into quarters lengthwise, then cut crosswise into 2-inch lengths.

3. Line a platter with the shredded cabbage. Arrange the broccoli, carrots, leeks, and sardines on cabbage. Pour the Warm Dill Dressing over the salad. Garnish with dill sprigs and serve.

Warm Dill Dressing

Makes about ⅔ cup

¼ cup olive oil

¼ cup water

2 ½ tablespoons apple-cider vinegar

1 large clove garlic, crushed through a press

¼ teaspoon freshly ground black pepper

2 to 3 tablespoons chopped fresh dill, or 2 teaspoons dried dill weed

Salt

In a small saucepan over low heat, combine the olive oil, vinegar, and garlic. Bring to a boil, whisking often. Remove the mixture from the heat and stir in the pepper and dill. Season with salt to taste.

Linguine with Fresh Fennel and Sardines

Makes 4 servings

1 large fresh fennel bulb

8 ounces whole-wheat linguine

2 tablespoons extra-virgin olive oil

2 cloves garlic, thinly sliced

¼ teaspoon crushed hot red pepper, or more to taste

2 tablespoons finely chopped flat-leaf parsley

Sea salt and freshly ground black pepper

2 cans (3.75 ounces each) Nordic brisling sardines

1. Trim the stems from the fennel bulb, reserving some of the dark green fronds for garnish. Cut the bulb in half and thinly slice.
2. In a large pot of boiling salted water, cook the linguine until al dente, about 12 minutes.
3. Meanwhile, heat the olive oil in a large skillet over medium-high heat. Add the fennel and cook, stirring occasionally, until softened and golden, about 10 minutes. Add the garlic and hot pepper and cook 1 to 2 minutes longer.
4. Remove ¾ cup of the pasta cooking water and set aside. Drain the pasta into a colander and immediately add to the fennel mixture in the skillet. Add the parsley and toss, adding as much of the reserved cooking water as needed to moisten the pasta. Season with salt and pepper to taste.
5. Divide the pasta among 4 pasta bowls or plates. Arrange the sardines on top, garnish with the fennel fronds, and serve.

Sardine Pasta Primavera

MAKES 4 SERVINGS

1 cup green beans cut into 1-inch pieces

1 cup sliced or slivered carrots

1 cup broccoli florets

1 cup sliced zucchini

12 ounces dried whole-wheat fettuccine, cooked until al dente, then well drained

⅓ cup plus 1 tablespoon extra-virgin olive oil

1 onion, chopped

2 large cloves garlic, minced

1 cup red and/or yellow bell pepper strips

¼ cup balsamic vinegar

2 tablespoons fresh thyme leaves or 2 teaspoons dried thyme

1 cup halved cherry tomatoes

Salt and freshly ground black pepper

2 cans (3.75 ounces each) Nordic brisling sardines in oil, drained

Grated Parmesan cheese

1. Bring a large pot of salted water to a boil. Add the green beans and carrot and cook for 2 minutes. Add the broccoli and zucchini; cook for 2 minute longer. With a slotted spoon, scoop out vegetables and drain in a colander Rinse briefly under cold running water, drain, and transfer to a large bow
2. Add pasta to same water and cook until al dente, about 10 minutes. Scoop out and reserve 1 cup pasta cooking water. Drain pasta into colander; toss with 1 tablespoon olive oil.
3. In a very large skillet or flameproof casserole, cook onion and garlic in remaining olive oil over medium-high heat, stirring occasionally, until the onion is soft and translucent, 3 to 5 minutes. Add the bell peppers and cook 1 to 2 minutes, or until just softened.
4. Add blanched vegetables, vinegar, thyme, tomatoes, and pasta to skillet. Cook, tossing and adding enough reserved cooking liquid to make a sauc until heated through. Season with salt and pepper to taste. Transfer to a large serving platter. Top with the sardines, sprinkle with the Parmesan, and serve.

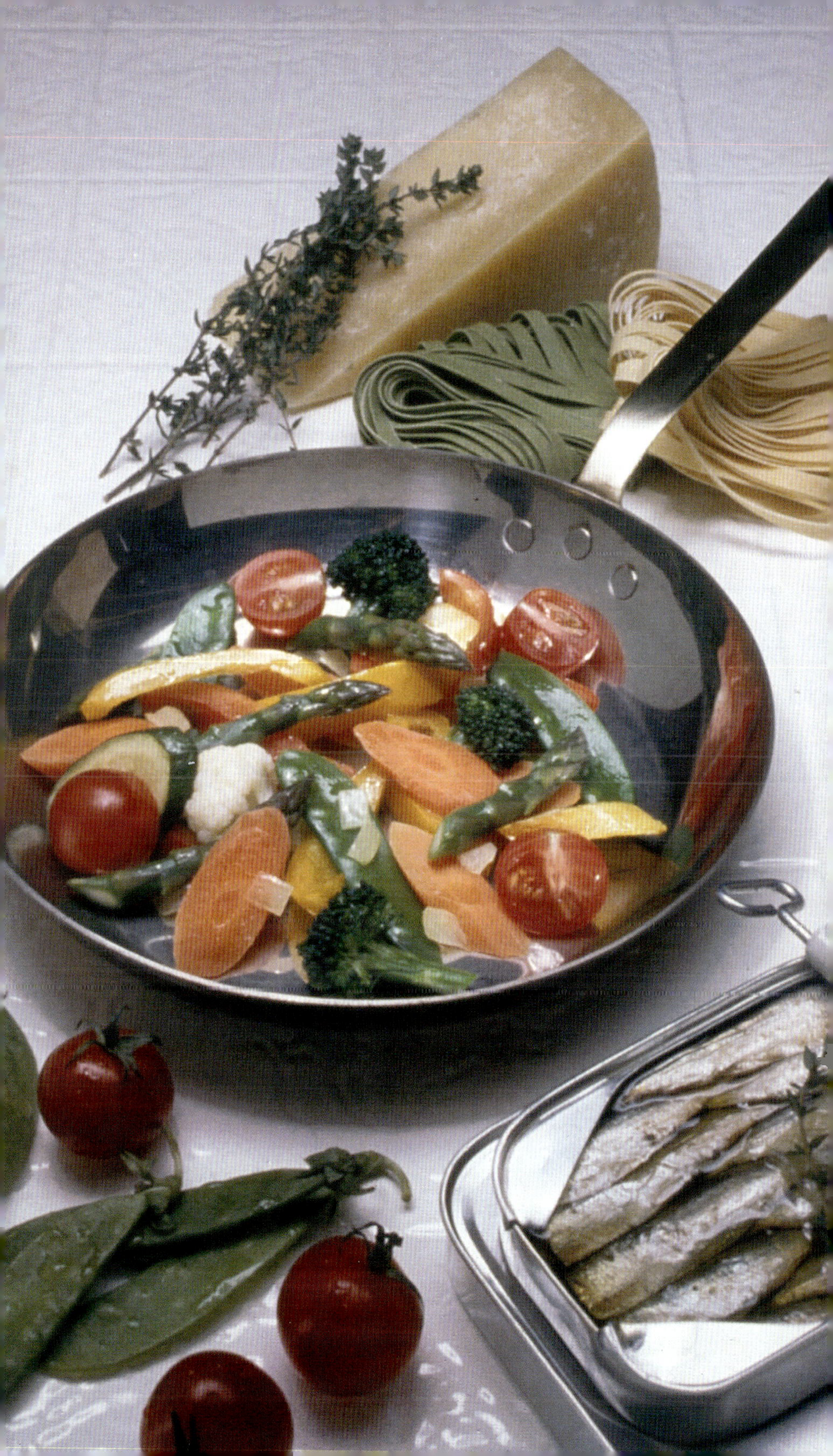

Cucumber Sardine Tea Sandwiches

Makes 16 sandwiches (4 appetizer servings)

6 tablespoons mayonnaise

1½ tablespoons drained capers

4 teaspoons Dijon mustard

1½ teaspoons minced fresh dill, or ½ teaspoon dried dill weed

2 whole-wheat pita breads (6 to 7 inches in diameter)

½ seedless cucumber, thinly sliced (about 30 slices)

1 can (3.75 ounces) Nordic brisling sardines in oil, drained

1. In a small bowl, mix the mayonnaise, capers, mustard and dill weed; set aside.
2. With a small sharp knife, cut the pitas around the edge; gently pull each bread apart to make circles.
3. Spread the inside of each circle with the mayonnaise mixture, dividing equally. Cover 2 of the circles with cucumber slices, then cover the cucumbers with half the sardines; press the sardines down with fork. Cover with the remaining bread circles, spread sides down. Lightly press on top circles.
4. With a large knife, cut each sandwich into 8 triangles. Serve immediately, or cover securely with plastic wrap and refrigerate for up to 2 hours before serving.

Whole-Wheat Pita Pizzas with Anchovies, Browned Onion, and Sweet Red Pepper

MAKES 4 SERVINGS

1 medium onion, thinly sliced

1½ tablespoons extra-virgin olive oil

4 whole-wheat pita pockets (about 6 inches in diameter)

4 ounces Manchego, Fontina, or Gruyère cheese, thinly sliced

1 can (2 ounces) anchovy fillets, drained

1 small red bell pepper, very thinly sliced

1. Heat the oven to 375°F, setting a rack in the top position. In a large nonstick skillet, cook the onion in 1 tablespoon of the olive oil with 2 tablespoons water over medium heat, covered, until softened, 2 to 3 minutes. Uncover, raise the heat to medium-high and cook, stirring often, until the onion is golden brown, 5 to 7 minutes longer.
2. Lay the pitas on a large baking sheet and brush lightly with the remaining olive oil. Bake for about 3 minutes to crisp slightly. Remove from the oven and let cool briefly.
3. Divide the cheese slices among the 4 pitas, covering to within ¼ inch of the edges of the bread. Scatter the browned onion over the cheese. Arrange the anchovies and red pepper slices decoratively on top.
4. Return the pizzas to the oven and bake for 5 minutes or until warmed through.

Pita Pockets with Lemony Hummus, Sardines, and Olives

Makes 4 servings

Brisling sardines are so mild and versatile that they blend with almost any seasoning. Here they head toward the Middle East with a creamy, lemony hummus and salty kalamata olives. Pass a bottle of hot sauce on the side.

4 whole-wheat pita pockets
2 large plum tomatoes, seeded and diced
⅓ cup seedless kalamata olives, coarsely chopped
¼ cup chopped scallions
1 tablespoon extra-virgin olive oil
¼ teaspoon crushed hot red pepper
Lemony Hummus (recipe on page 83)
2 cans (3.75 ounces each) Nordic brisling sardines
1½ cups shredded romaine or iceberg lettuce

1. Cut the top quarter or third off the pita breads and gently open them up to make pockets.
2. In a medium-size bowl, combine the tomatoes, olives, and scallions. Toss with the olive oil and hot pepper.
3. Spoon 2 tablespoons hummus into each pita pocket. Divide the tomato-olive mixture among the pockets. Tuck in the sardines and top with the lettuce. Serve at once.

Lemony Hummus

MAKES ABOUT 1 CUP

1 small can (9 ounces) chickpeas

1 ½ tablespoons tahini (Middle Eastern sesame paste)

¾ teaspoon ground cumin

1 garlic clove, crushed through a press

1 lemon

2 tablespoons fruity extra-virgin olive oil

Salt and cayenne pepper

1. Drain the chickpeas into a colander. Rinse well under cold running water and drain, shaking the colander to remove most of the moisture.
2. In a food processor, combine the chickpeas, tahini, cumin, and garlic. Grate about ½ teaspoon of the lemon zest into the processor. Cut the lemon in half and squeeze in the juice, making sure to remove all seeds. Puree until smooth.
3. With the machine on, add the olive oil through the feed tube. Also add 3 to 4 tablespoons hot water, or enough to thin the hummus to the consistency of sour cream. Season with salt and cayenne to taste.

Deviled Sardine Spread

MAKES ABOUT ¾ CUP

If you prepare this spread in advance, it will continue to get hotter as the mustard develops flavor over time, which is perfect for those who like it hot. Season with salt and pepper to taste and serve with crisp toasts or rice crackers.

2 cans (3.75 ounces each) Nordic brisling sardines, drained

2 tablespoons fresh lemon juice

2 teaspoons grated onion

1 teaspoon powdered mustard

½ teaspoon Tabasco sauce

2 teaspoons low-fat mayonnaise

Salt and freshly ground black pepper

Mash the sardines with a fork until crushed to a coarse paste. Add the lemon juice, onion, mustard, Tabasco sauce, and mayonnaise. Blend well. Season with salt and pepper to taste.

Omega Spread

MAKES ABOUT ½ CUP

1 can (3.75 ounces) Nordic brisling sardines, drained

1 tablespoon minced onion

¼ cup finely chopped celery

2 tablespoons low-fat mayonnaise

½ teaspoon Dijon mustard

½ teaspoon fresh lemon juice

2 tablespoons sweet relish (optional)

In a small bowl, mash sardines and combine with the rest of the ingredients. Blend well. Serve with high-fiber crackers, stuffed into celery sticks, or on bread as a sandwich, with lettuce and tomato.

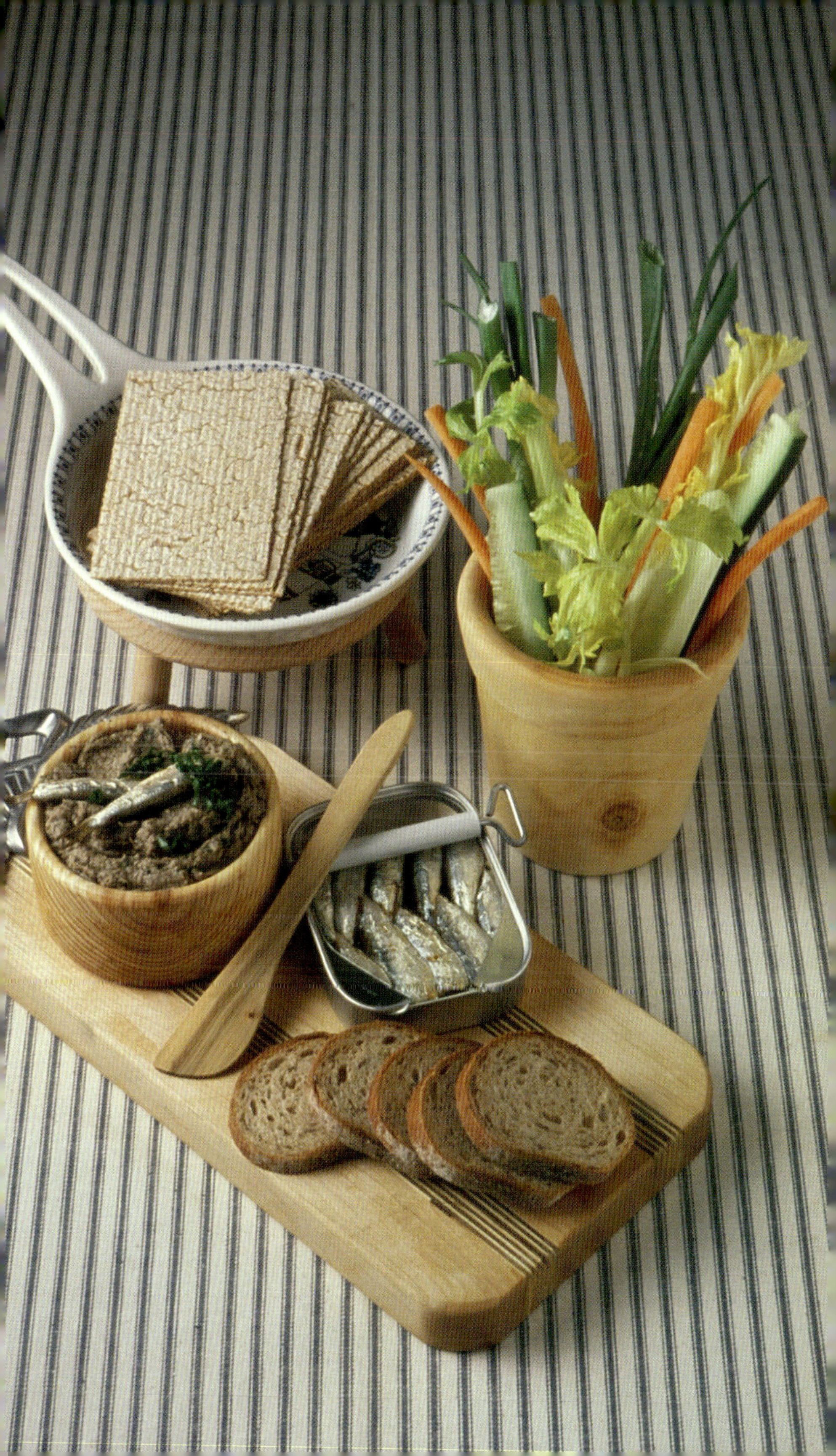

The recipes on the next 8 pages contain no sardines, but are essential to the weight-loss meal plan on pages 50–57.

Carrot-Cabbage Slaw

Makes ⅔ cup

1 small carrot, peeled

½-inch wedge of cabbage

1 ½ tablespoons apple-cider vinegar

Salt and freshly ground pepper

Shred the carrot and cabbage in a food processor or on a box grater. Toss with the vinegar and season with salt and pepper to taste. Eat right away, or marinate in a resealable plastic bag for added flavor.

Savory Spinach Dip

Makes about 1¾ cups

Use this savory blend as a dip for carrots, cucumbers, zucchini or high-fiber crackers when entertaining or anytime you need a satisfying snack.

1 cup (8 ounces) nonfat sour cream or plain yogurt

⅔ envelope vegetable soup mix

½ (10-ounce) package frozen chopped spinach, thawed and squeezed dry

⅓ cup finely chopped water chestnuts (optional)

In a small bowl, stir together the sour cream or yogurt and soup mix. Add the spinach and water chestnuts. Blend well. Cover and refrigerate until ready to eat.

Vinaigrette

Makes 3/4 cup (12 tablespoons)

Use your best, most flavorful cold-pressed olive oil for this simple dressing. If you're on the diet, allow 1 or 2 tablespoons per serving, according to the menu plan. Store leftovers in a tightly covered jar in the refrigerator for up to a week.

1/2 cup extra-virgin olive oil
1/4 cup fresh lemon juice
1/2 teaspoon salt
1/4 teaspoon freshly ground black pepper

In a jar with a tight-fitting lid, combine all the ingredients. Shake vigorously to blend, about 15 seconds.

Roasted Chicken Lettuce Wraps

Makes 1 Serving

3 romaine lettuce leaves
4 ounces skinned roasted chicken, diced
1/4 cup chopped cucumbers
2 tablespoons chopped bell peppers
1 ounce shredded low-fat cheese
1 tablespoon salsa, for dipping

Lay one lettuce leaf on a plate. Top with one-third each of the chicken, cucumber, and pepper. Sprinkle with the cheese and roll up. Repeat with the remaining lettuce leaves and serve with salsa on the side.

Keri's Broiled Chicken

Makes 6 to 8 Servings

Here you get the satisfaction of roast chicken on the bone without the added fat from skin. This recipe makes enough for a family meal.

4 chicken breasts on the bone (about 6 ounces), skin removed

½ cup low-sodium chicken broth, plus more for basting

1 tablespoon Worcestershire sauce, plus more for basting

Salt, freshly ground black pepper, and paprika

Onion and/or garlic powder

1. Set the oven rack about 6 inches from heat source and heat the broiler. Place the chicken breasts in a shallow broiling pan. Pour the broth and Worcestershire sauce over chicken. Season to taste with salt, pepper, paprika, and onion and/or garlic powder.
2. Broil the chicken until lightly browned on top, 8 to 10 minutes. Turn the chicken over and baste with pan juices. Broil second side until lightly browned, 8 to 10 minutes longer. If the pan juices have evaporated, baste with the additional broth and Worcestershire.
3. Cover the chicken loosely with aluminum foil, turn off the heat, and let the chicken rest in the hot oven for 5 minutes longer, or until it is white in the center, but still juicy. Serve with the pan juices.

Maple-Walnut Baked Apple

Makes 1 Serving

1 baking apple, cored

1 small dried fig, chopped

1 teaspoon chopped walnuts

1 teaspoon maple syrup

Cinnamon

Heat oven to 350°F. Place the apple in a baking pan and fill the core with chopped fig and walnuts. Drizzle maple syrup into center. Dust the apple with cinnamon. Pour ¾ cup hot water over the apple. Bake, basting often, until apple is tender, 40 to 50 minutes.

Grilled Pineapple Slices

Makes 6 to 8 Servings

1 whole ripe pineapple

1 tablespoon maple syrup or honey

Grated nutmeg

Cut off the top and bottom of the pineapple, then slice off the outer skin and prickly "eyes," leaving the whole pineapple. Turn the fruit on its side and cut into ½-inch rounds. Brush each slice lightly with maple syrup. Dust the pineapple slices lightly with nutmeg. Grill or broil 2 to 4 minutes per side, until the fruit is hot and lightly browned. Serve warm.

Oatmeal Pancake

Makes 1 Serving

½ cup oatmeal flakes

½ cup egg whites

1 teaspoon maple syrup

In a small bowl, stir together the oatmeal and egg whites. Heat a nonstick pan over medium-high heat until hot. Pour the oatmeal mixture into the pan and cook, turning once, until golden. Serve hot with maple syrup.

Spinach Omelet with Tomatoes and Parmesan Cheese

Makes 1 Serving

¼ cup chopped spinach

¼ cup diced tomatoes

3 egg whites, beaten until frothy

1 tablespoon grated Parmesan cheese

2 tablespoons Vinaigrette (page 87)

Heat a nonstick pan over medium heat until hot. Add the spinach and the tomatoes and sauté for 30 seconds; add the eggs. As the eggs set around the edge of the skillet, pull the cooked portions toward the center with a heatproof spatula, letting raw egg flow around and underneath. Repeat until the eggs are partially set, about 1 minute, then sprinkle with cheese. Fold the omelet over and continue cooking for 30 seconds longer. Serve hot with vinaigrette on the side.

Scrambled Egg with Smoked Salmon

Makes 1 Serving

1 egg, beaten

2 ounces smoked salmon

Heat a nonstick pan over medium-high heat until hot. Add salmon and sauté for 30 seconds. Add the egg and scramble until it is cooked to the desired doneness.

Cheddar-Broccoli Omelet

Makes 1 Serving

3 egg whites, beaten until frothy

¼ cup chopped cooked broccoli

1 ounce reduced-fat Cheddar cheese

Heat a nonstick pan over medium heat until hot. Add the broccoli and sauté for 30 seconds; add the eggs. As the eggs set around the edge of the skillet, pull the cooked portions toward the center with a heatproof spatula, letting raw egg flow around and underneath. Repeat until the eggs are partially set, about 1 minute, then sprinkle with cheese. Fold the omelet over and continue cooking for 30 seconds longer. Serve hot.

French Toast

Makes 1 Serving

1 slice whole wheat bread

2 egg whites, beaten until frothy

Cinnamon

In a small casserole dish, soak the bread in the egg whites for 1 minute. Heat a nonstick pan over medium heat until hot. Add the soaked bread and cook, turning once, until golden brown on both sides, about 3 minutes. Sprinkle with cinnamon and serve.

Breakfast Burrito

½ cup nonfat plain yogurt

½ cup salsa

2 egg whites

1 whole egg

¼ cup sliced red bell pepper

1 high-fiber tortilla

1. In a small bowl, stir together the yogurt and salsa; set aside. In a second small bowl, whisk together the egg whites and whole egg.
2. Heat a small nonstick pan over medium heat until hot; add the red pepper slices and sauté for 30 seconds. Pour the eggs over the peppers and scramble until the mixture is cooked to the desired doneness. Spoon the egg mixture into the tortilla and roll up into a burrito.

Yogurt Parfait

Makes 1 Serving

- 1/4 cup high-fiber cereal
- 1 tablespoon wheat germ
- 1 tablespoon ground flaxseeds
- 1 cup sliced strawberries
- 1 cup nonfat plain yogurt
- Cinnamon

In a small bowl, stir together the cereal, wheat germ, and flaxseeds. In a parfait glass or tall drinking glass, add a layer of strawberries, topped with a layer of yogurt and then a layer of the cereal mixture, repeating layers until all the ingredients have been used. Sprinkle with cinnamon and serve.

The following recipes all contain Nordic brisling sardines, so not only are they rich in omega-3s; they are delicious. Enjoy!

Pizza from the Pantry

Makes 1 large pizza (4 servings)

2 tablespoons olive oil

4 cloves garlic, thinly sliced

1 tablespoon fresh oregano leaves, or 1 teaspoon dried oregano

1 tablespoon fresh rosemary leaves, or 1 teaspoon dried rosemary

1 package (10 ounces) prepared refrigerated pizza dough

2/3 cup sliced pitted black olives

1/2 cup roasted red bell pepper strips

3/4 cup shredded Fontina cheese

1 can (3.75 ounces) Nordic brisling sardines in oil, drained

1. Heat oven to 425°F. In a small bowl, combine the oil, garlic, oregano, and rosemary; set aside. Pat the dough into a greased 12-inch round pizza pan or 9 x 13-inch baking pan. Prick all over with a fork. Brush the dough with seasoned oil. Scatter the olives and pepper strips over the dough and sprinkle with cheese.
2. Bake the pizza for 18 to 20 minutes or until crust is golden brown and cheese is bubbly. Remove pizza from the oven, and arrange the sardines on top. Serve hot.

Nordic Pizza

Makes two 12-inch pizzas (8 servings)

1 package (13-3/4 ounces) pizza-dough mix (that calls for 1 egg)

½ teaspoon oregano

Extra-virgin olive oil

2 jars (8 ounces each) pizza sauce

8 ounces shredded mozzarella, Monterey Jack, or Cheddar cheese (about 2 to 3 cups)

Sliced fresh mushrooms

2 cans (3.75 ounces each) Nordic brisling sardines, drained

1 green bell pepper, cut into thin rings

Halved cherry tomatoes

Grated Parmesan cheese

1. Prepare the dough mix, as package directs, adding the oregano with the egg. Knead on a floured board until smooth and elastic, about 5 minutes. Cover and let rise in a warm place until doubled in bulk, about 45 minutes. Punch down. Divide the dough in half. Roll out to fit 2 lightly oiled 12-inch pizza pans*. Prick several times with fork. Brush with the olive oil. Let rise 20 minutes.
2. About 30 minutes before serving, spread the tomato sauce evenly over pizza crusts. Sprinkle the cheese over the sauce. Arrange the mushroom slices and sardines in rings around the edge.
3. Heat oven to 425°F. Bake for 10 minutes. Remove the pizzas from the oven; arrange the green pepper rings and halved cherry tomatoes decoratively in center of each pizza. Sprinkle each pizza with Parmesan cheese. Return to the oven and bake for 5 to 10 minutes longer.

** Jelly-roll pans or baking sheets can be used in place of pizza pans. Roll dough out to rectangles to fit, and build up the sides slightly after fitting it into pan.*

Anchovy Bruschetta with Toasted Walnuts

Makes 4 first-course servings

12 anchovy fillets, drained

2 teaspoons Dijon mustard

1 teaspoon coarsely ground black pepper

3 ½ tablespoons extra-virgin olive oil

2 tablespoons unsalted butter, at room temperature

1 clove garlic, finely minced

¼ cup chopped walnuts

4 thick slices crusty whole-grain bread

1. Using a fork, mash the anchovies in a small bowl. In another small bowl, whisk together the mustard, pepper, 2 tablespoons of the olive oil, butter, and minced garlic. Add to the anchovies and mix to form a paste.
2. Heat the remaining 1½ tablespoons olive oil in a small skillet. Add the walnuts and sauté over medium heat until lightly toasted, 3 to 5 minutes.
3. Toast the bread. Spread the anchovy mixture over each slice while still warm. Top with toasted walnuts. Serve immediately.

Avocado and Sardine Canapés

Makes 12 pieces

To make these easy appetizers, slices of bread are quartered on the diagonal. If you leave them whole or simply cut them in half, they can be enjoyed as open-faced sandwiches instead.

3 slices high-fiber or multigrain bread, preferably thinly sliced

1 ½ tablespoons extra-virgin olive oil

2 teaspoons fresh lemon juice

2 teaspoons champagne or white-wine vinegar

Salt and freshly ground black pepper

1 Hass avocado

1 tablespoon minced cilantro or parsley, plus small sprigs for garnish

1 ½ teaspoons minced shallot

1 can (3.75 ounces) Nordic brisling sardines, drained

1. Toast the bread until crisp.
2. In a small bowl, whisk together the olive oil, lemon juice, and vinegar. Season with salt and pepper to taste.
3. Cut the avocado lengthwise in half around the pit. Twist to separate the 2 halves; remove the pit. Scoop out the avocado with a large spoon and cut into small dice. Toss the diced avocado with half the vinaigrette. Add the cilantro and shallot and toss to mix.
4. Divide the avocado mixture among the 4 slices of toast. Cut each slice on the diagonal into 4 triangles. Top each triangle with 1 or 2 sardines. Drizzle the remaining vinaigrette over the top and garnish each with a small sprig of cilantro.

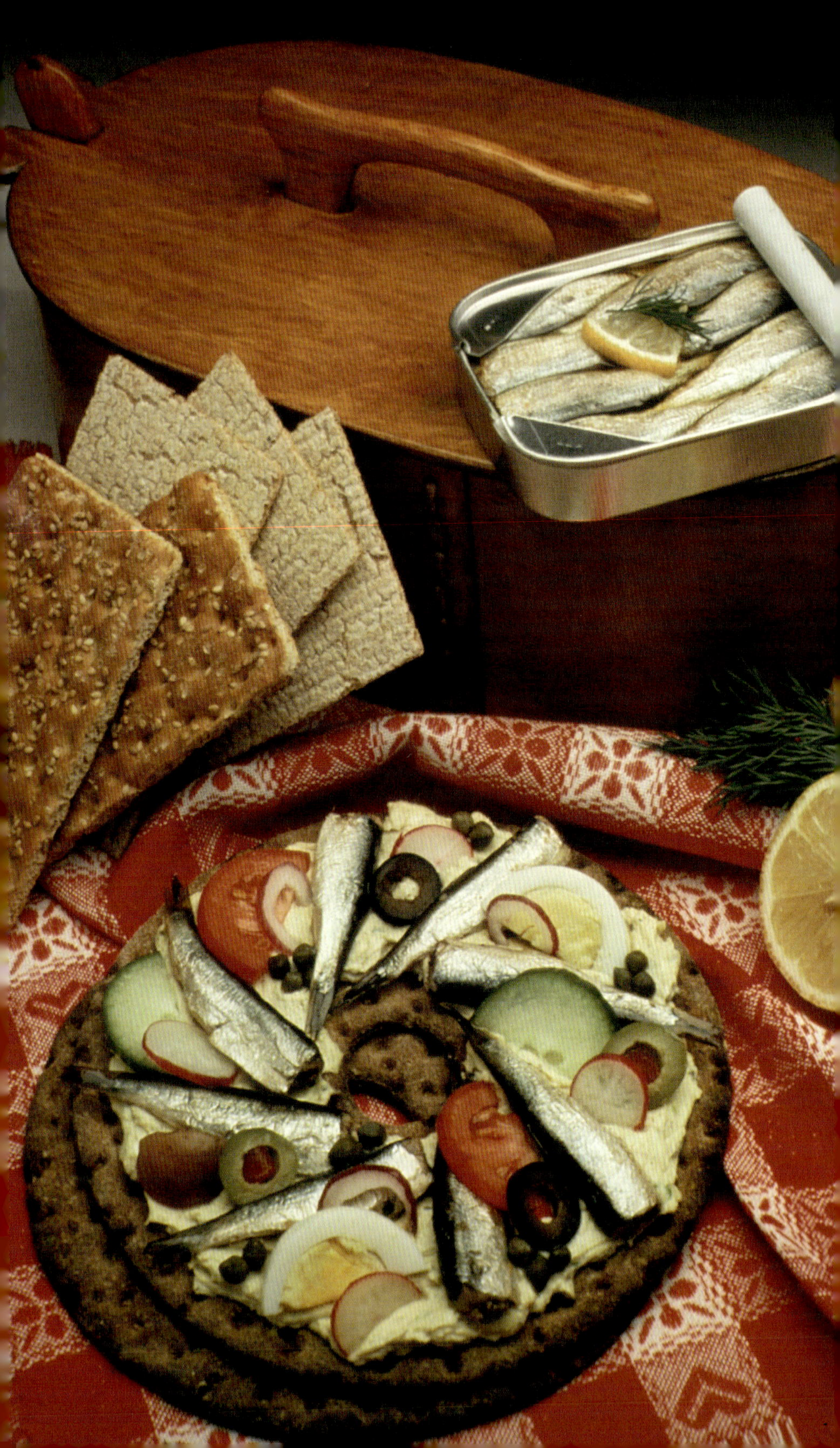

Spring Sardine Knäckebröd

MAKES 8 TO 10 APPETIZER SERVINGS OR 4 MAIN-DISH SERVINGS

1 package (8 ounces) reduced-fat cream cheese (Neufchâtel), softened

1 tablespoon Dijon mustard

1 tablespoon reduced-calorie mayonnaise

1 tablespoon finely chopped shallots

2 teaspoons fresh lemon juice

2 cans (3.75 ounces each) Nordic brisling sardines in oil, drained

1 round Scandinavian knäckebröd cracker (about 10 inches in diameter)*

1½ to 2 cups toppings of your choice (sliced tomatoes, cucumber, radishes, red onion, red and green bell pepper, ripe and green olives, hard-cooked eggs, cooked tiny red potatoes, capers, dill sprigs, parsley sprigs)

Lemon wedges

1. In bowl, blend together cream cheese, mustard, mayonnaise, shallots, lemon juice, and ½ can sardines. Spread over knäckebröd.
2. Arrange toppings and the remaining sardines on top. Using a chef's knife, cut knäckebröd into serving pieces. Serve immediately with lemon wedges on the side.

** Knäckebröd is available in the cracker or gourmet sections of most supermarkets. Smaller knäckebröd or other crisp rye crackers can be substituted.*

Asparagus and Sardine Toasts

Makes 2 servings

3 tablespoons chopped parsley

2 teaspoons minced garlic

1 teaspoon grated lemon zest

2 tablespoons extra-virgin olive oil

4 slices French bread (½-inch thick), toasted

16 asparagus tips, cooked until crisp-tender and drained

2 cans (3.75 ounces each) Nordic brisling sardines in oil, drained

Halved cherry tomatoes, for garnish

1. In a small bowl, mix the parsley, garlic, and lemon zest; set aside. Brush the toast with olive oil.
2. On each slice of toast, arrange 4 asparagus tips and ½ can of sardines. Sprinkle with the parsley mixture and garnish with the cherry tomatoes.

Sardine Spread with Olives, Roasted Peppers, and Pine Nuts

MAKES ABOUT 1½ CUPS

2 cans (3.75 ounces each) Nordic brisling sardines in oil, drained, a few reserved for garnish

¼ cup sliced ripe and/or pimiento-stuffed olives

¼ cup chopped roasted red peppers or pimientos

¼ cup chopped red onion

2 cloves garlic, crushed through a press

2 tablespoons mayonnaise

2 tablespoons toasted pine nuts, plus more for garnish

1 tablespoon fresh lemon juice

1½ teaspoons dried oregano

Put sardines (except for those reserved) in a bowl with all the remaining ingredients and mix with a fork to blend thoroughly. Pack into a small bowl or crock or into a large red pepper. Garnish with the reserved whole sardines, additional olives slices and pine nuts. Serve with crackers and bread.

Celeste Holm's Norwegian Sardine Spread

Makes about 1 cup

2 cans (3.75 ounces each) Nordic brisling sardines packed in oil, drained

3 tablespoons plain yogurt

3 tablespoons mayonnaise

1½ teaspoons soy sauce

1½ teaspoons fresh lemon juice

Fresh parsley or dill sprigs, for garnish

Assorted breads, crackers, and raw vegetables, for serving

1. In a small bowl, lightly mash the sardines with a fork. Add the yogurt, mayonnaise, soy sauce, and lemon juice. Blend well.
2. To serve, spoon the spread into a serving bowl and garnish with parsley or dill. Serve chilled or at room temperature as a spread or dip for assorted crackers and fresh vegetables.

Sardine Pâté

Makes about 2 cups

2 cans (3.75 ounces each) Nordic brisling sardines in oil, drained

2 hard-cooked eggs

4 tablespoons butter, softened

2 tablespoons mayonnaise

1½ tablespoons fresh lime juice

1 teaspoon Dijon mustard

¼ cup chopped celery

2 tablespoons chopped parsley, plus more for garnish

Salt and freshly ground black pepper

Crackers or whole-grain bread, for serving

1. Combine the sardines, eggs, butter, mayonnaise, lime juice, and mustard in a food processor or electric blender; blend until smooth. Stir in the celery and parsley.
2. To serve, spoon the pâté into a serving bowl or small crock. Cover and refrigerate until chilled. Garnish with additional chopped parsley. Serve pâté with cheese and crackers.

Sardine Tostadas with Avocado Salsa

Makes 6 appetizer servings

6 corn tortillas

1½ cups shredded lettuce

6 ounces Monterey Jack cheese, shredded (about 1½ cups)

2 ripe plum tomatoes, seeded and finely diced (1 cup)

Avocado Salsa (recipe follows)

3 cans (3.75 ounces each) Nordic brisling sardines in olive oil or in salsa, drained

½ cup sour cream

Sprigs of cilantro, for garnish

1. Heat the oven to 250°F. Place the tortillas directly on the oven rack and toast for 4 to 5 minutes or until crisp.
2. Layer the lettuce, cheese, tomatoes, and Avocado Salsa on each tortilla, dividing equally. Top with the sardines and a small dollop of sour cream. Garnish with cilantro.

Avocado Salsa

1 small ripe avocado, preferably Hass

⅓ cup finely chopped white onion

2 tablespoons chopped cilantro (optional)

½ jalapeño pepper, seeds removed and minced

1 tablespoon lemon juice

Salt

In a small bowl, mash the avocado slightly with a fork. Add onion, cilantro, jalapeño, and lemon juice; stir to combine. Season with salt to taste.

Pimiento Cheese–Sardine Wraps

Makes 4 servings

4 ounces fat-free soft cream cheese

½ cup diced pimiento or roasted red pepper

1 tablespoon chopped fresh dill or parsley

½ teaspoon white-wine vinegar

Salt and hot paprika or cayenne pepper

4 whole-wheat tortillas

2 cans (3.75 ounces each) Nordic brisling sardines, drained

1. In a small bowl, blend together the cream cheese, pimiento, dill, and vinegar. Season with salt and hot paprika or cayenne to taste.
2. Spoon a line of pimiento cheese down one side of each tortilla. Top with the sardines. Roll up and cut diagonally in half.

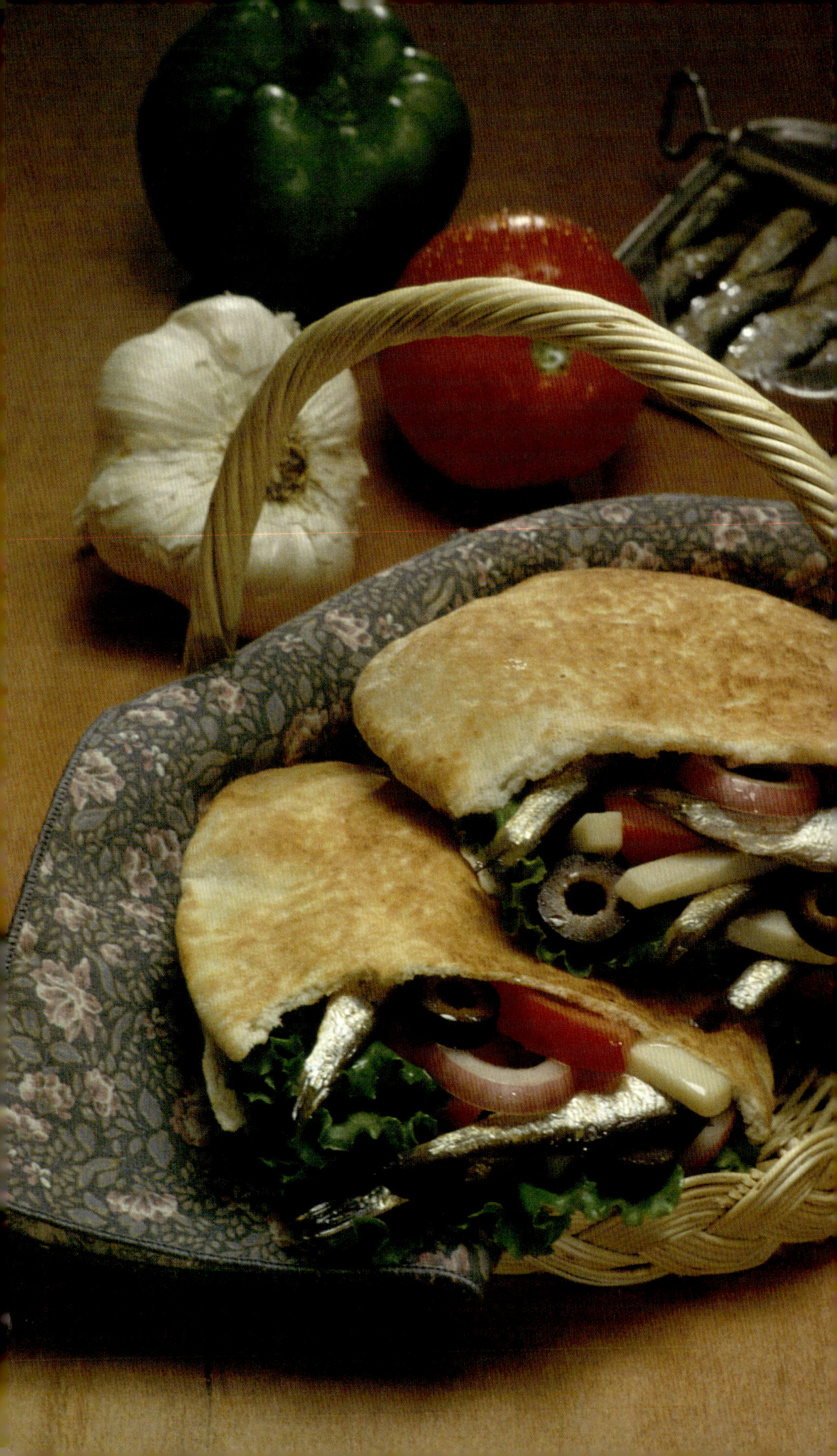

Sardine and Olive Antipasto Sandwiches

Makes 8 sandwiches (4 servings)

1 cup sliced pitted black olives

½ cup coarsely chopped artichoke hearts

½ cup roasted red pepper strips

½ cup slivered Provolone cheese

⅓ cup thinly sliced red onion

1 medium tomato, cut into thin wedges

2 tablespoons red-wine vinegar

1 tablespoon extra-virgin olive oil

2 cloves garlic, minced

1 teaspoon dried oregano

Salt and pepper

2 cans (3.75 ounces each) Nordic brisling sardines in oil, drained

4 whole-wheat pita breads (about 6 inches in diameter)

8 small lettuce leaves

In a large bowl, combine all ingredients except the sardines, pita breads, and lettuce. Toss to mix. Add the sardines; toss lightly. Halve the breads and open the pockets. Line one side of each pocket with lettuce; spoon about ½ cup of the sardine mixture into each. Serve at room temperature.

Hearty Sardine Sandwiches

Makes 4 servings

1 cup chopped cucumber

½ cup shredded carrot

3 tablespoons sliced shallots

1½ teaspoons mustard seeds

1½ tablespoons white-wine vinegar

Salt

2 tablespoons extra-virgin olive oil

1 small clove garlic, crushed through a press

8 slices whole grain bread

Lettuce or spinach leaves

2 cans (3.75 ounces each) Nordic brisling sardines in oil, drained

1. In a small bowl, combine the cucumber, carrot, shallots, mustard seeds, and vinegar. Season with salt to taste.
2. Heat the oven to 425°F. In another small bowl, combine oil and garlic; brush on one side of each bread slice. Place the bread directly on the oven rack. Bake until lightly browned, 5 to 10 minutes.
3. For each sandwich, arrange the lettuce and ½ can of the sardines on a slice of toast and top with a generous ¼ cup of the cucumber mixture. Top with another slice of toast. Press lightly and cut in half before serving.

Tangy Sardine Sandwich with Horseradish, Capers, and Dill

MAKES 4 SERVINGS

¼ cup non-fat yogurt

1 tablespoon minced red onion

1 to 2 tablespoons chopped fresh dill

1 tablespoon tiny nonpareil capers

2 teaspoons prepared white horseradish

Freshly ground black pepper

4 whole-wheat sandwich rolls, cut in half

2 cans (3.75 ounces each) Nordic brisling sardines, drained

1 large tomato, sliced

4 lettuce leaves

1. In a small bowl, combine the yogurt, onion, dill, capers, horseradish, and pepper to taste. Spread the mixture over the halved rolls.
2. Layer the sardines, tomato slices, and lettuce on half of each roll and top with the other half.

Hot Sardine Sandwiches with Olive Spread

MAKES 4 SERVINGS

½ cup pimiento-stuffed green olives, drained

1½ tablespoons mayonnaise

¼ teaspoon dried dill weed

Freshly ground black pepper

8 slices light rye bread

4 ounces Swiss or Jarlsberg cheese, thinly sliced

2 medium tomatoes, sliced

1 small red onion, thinly sliced

2 cans (3.75 ounces each) Nordic brisling sardines in oil, drained

1. To make the olive spread, combine the olives, mayonnaise, and dill in a food processor or blender. Pulse on and off until the olives are very finely chopped. Season with pepper to taste.
2. Lightly toast the bread slices and place them on a baking sheet; cover 4 slices with cheese and 4 slices with the olive mixture, dividing equally. Broil until the cheese is melted.
3. For each sandwich, layer a cheese-covered slice of bread with tomato slices, onion slices, and ½ can of sardines. Top with an olive-spread slice. Cut in half; serve warm.

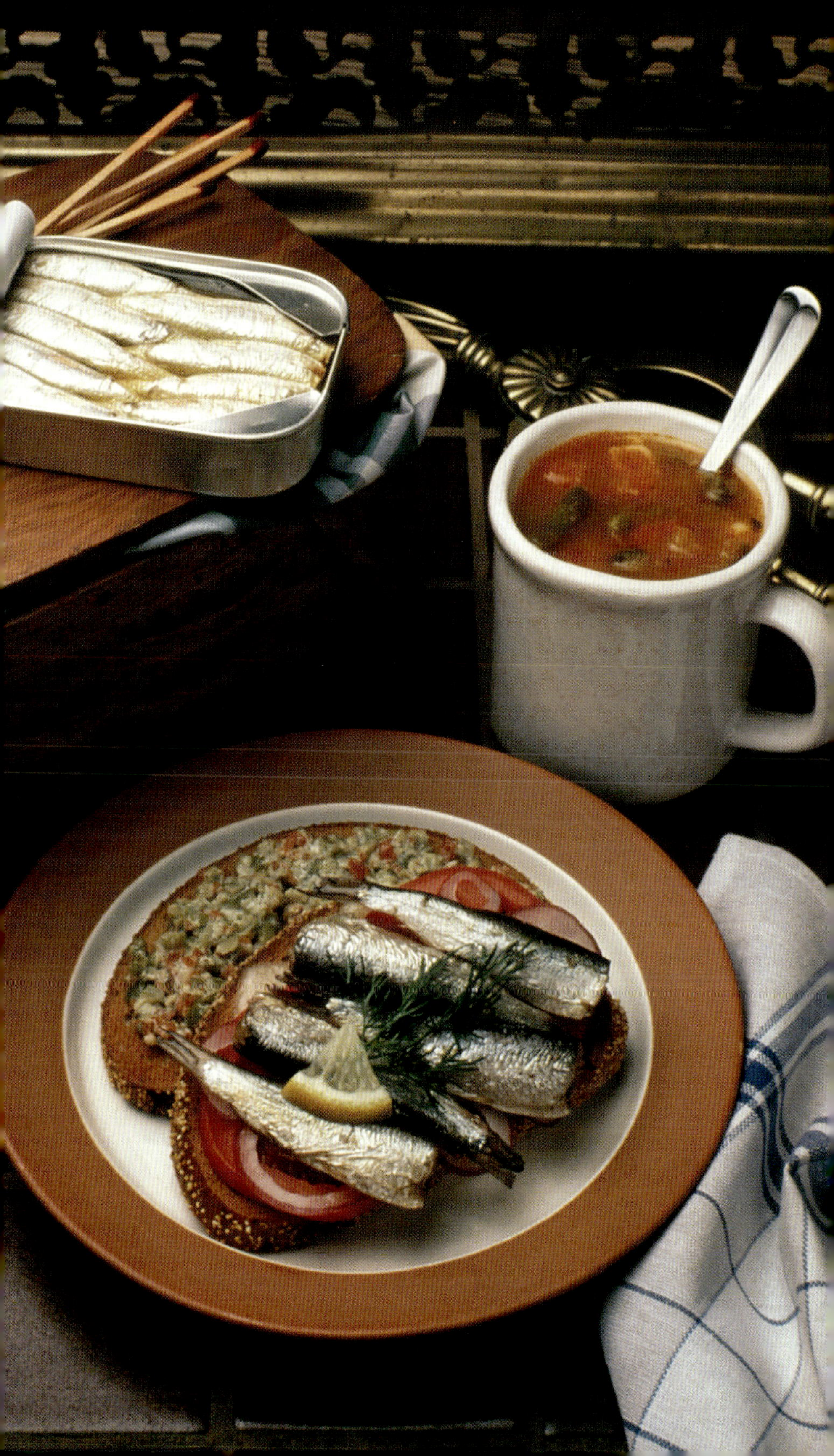

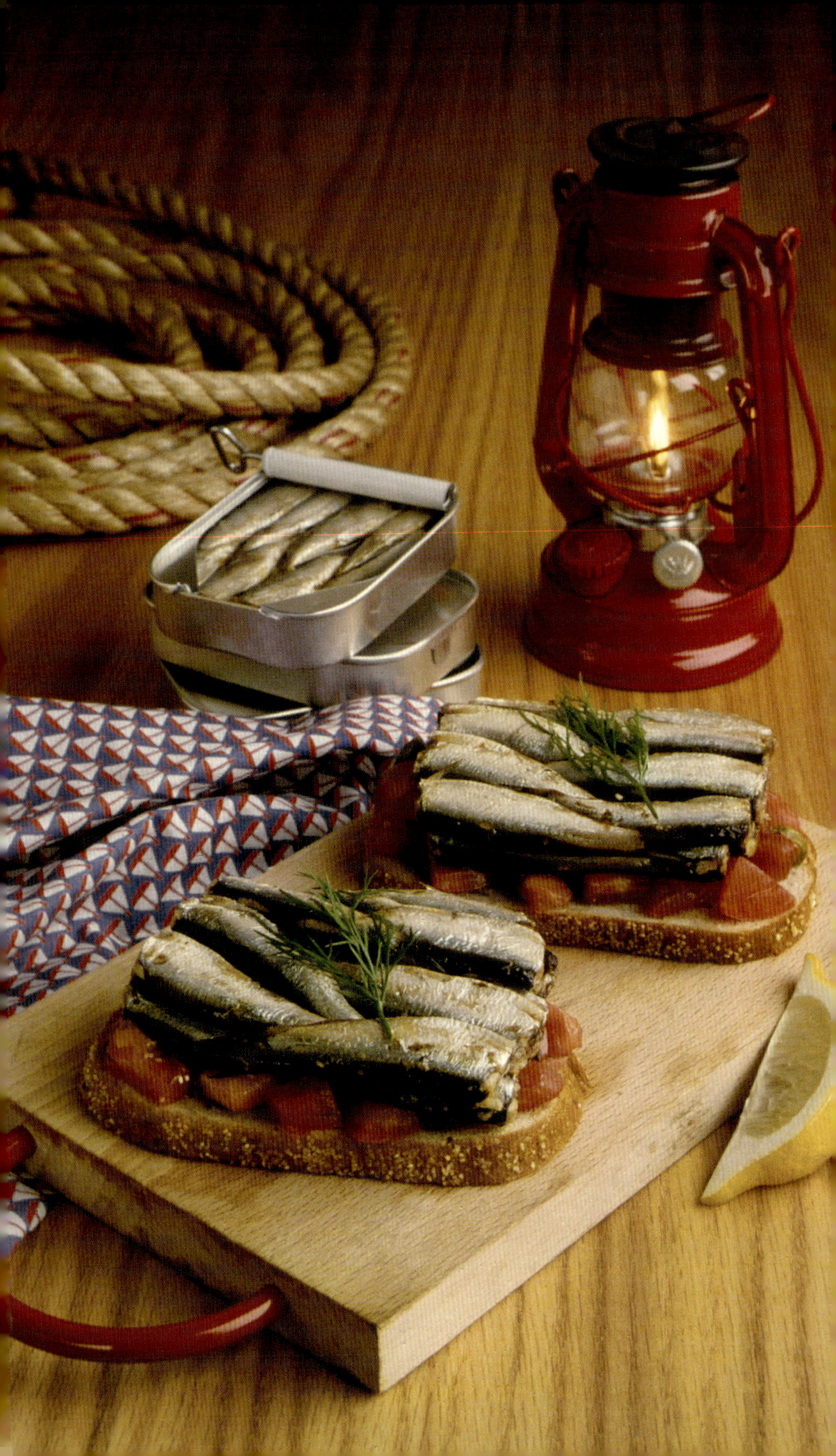

High Seas Sardine Sandwiches

Makes 4 servings

2 cups chopped tomatoes

1 tablespoon extra-virgin olive oil

2 cloves garlic, minced

1 tablespoon capers, drained

1 teaspoon chopped oregano or ¼ teaspoon dried oregano

Salt and pepper, to taste

Hot pepper sauce, to taste

4 slices Italian bread

4 cans (3.75 ounces each) Nordic brisling sardines in oil, drained

Lemon wedges, for garnish

1. In a large nonstick skillet, sauté the tomatoes in olive oil until they soften and the liquid evaporates, 5 to 10 minutes. Add the garlic, capers, and oregano. Cook, stirring, for 1 minute longer. Remove from heat. Season tomato puree with salt, pepper, and hot sauce. Let cool, then cover and refrigerate for at least 1 hour or up to 24 hours.
2. To assemble each sandwich, spread ¼ of the tomato puree over each bread slice. Top each slice with 1 can of sardines. Garnish with dill sprigs and lemon wedges.

Dilled Beet and Potato Salad with Sardines and Green Apple

Makes 4 servings

To turn this pretty appetizer into a main-course salad, serve on a bed of greens and accompany with rye crisps or whole grain bread.

3 medium beets

3 medium-large Yukon Gold potatoes

1 large Granny Smith apple

1 medium shallot, minced

¼ teaspoon sea salt

¼ cup red-wine or apple-cider vinegar

¼ cup extra-virgin olive oil

½ teaspoon sugar

Freshly ground black pepper

⅓ cup plus 1 tablespoon coarsely chopped fresh dill

2 cans (3.75 ounces each) Nordic brisling sardines, drained

1. Heat the oven to 400°F. Cut the green leaves off the beets, leaving about 1 inch of stem; rinse well. Wrap each beet in aluminum foil and roast in the oven for 1 to 1½ hours, or until the beet gives slightly when pressed. Unwrap and let cool. Cut off the tops, trim the root, and rub off the skin, which will come off easily. Cut the beets into ⅜-inch dice.

2. Meanwhile, in a pot of boiling water, cook the potatoes until tender, about 25 minutes. Rinse in cold water until cool enough to handle. Peel off the skin and cut the potato into ⅜-inch dice. Peel the apple and cut into ¼-inch dice.

3. Place the shallot in a large bowl. Sprinkle with the salt and vinegar; let stand for a minute or two. Whisk in the olive oil, sugar, and pepper.

4. Add the beets, potatoes, apple, and ⅓ cup of the dill. Toss to mix. Serve at once or cover and refrigerate for up to 2 days. When ready to serve, spoon the salad onto a platter or divide among plates. Arrange the sardines on top and garnish with the remaining dill.

Nordic Sea Salad

Makes 4 servings

2 cans (3.75 ounces each) Nordic brisling sardines in oil, drained

3 tablespoons nonfat yogurt

1½ tablespoons lemon juice

1 tablespoon prepared white horseradish

⅓ cup thinly sliced celery

⅓ cup thinly sliced scallions

Butter lettuce, romaine, or spinach leaves with stems removed

2 hard-cooked eggs, sliced

Salt

Crackers, breadsticks, or rye bread, for serving

1. Reserve a few sardines for garnish. In a small bowl, mix the remaining sardines with the yogurt, lemon juice, and horseradish to blend well, breaking up the fish as little as possible. Add the celery and scallions and mix lightly to combine evenly. Season with salt to taste. Cover and refrigerate until chilled.
2. Just before serving, make a bed of greens around the edge of a small platter and top with the sardine salad. Garnish with reserved whole sardines and hard-cooked egg slices. Serve with crackers, breadsticks, or rye bread.

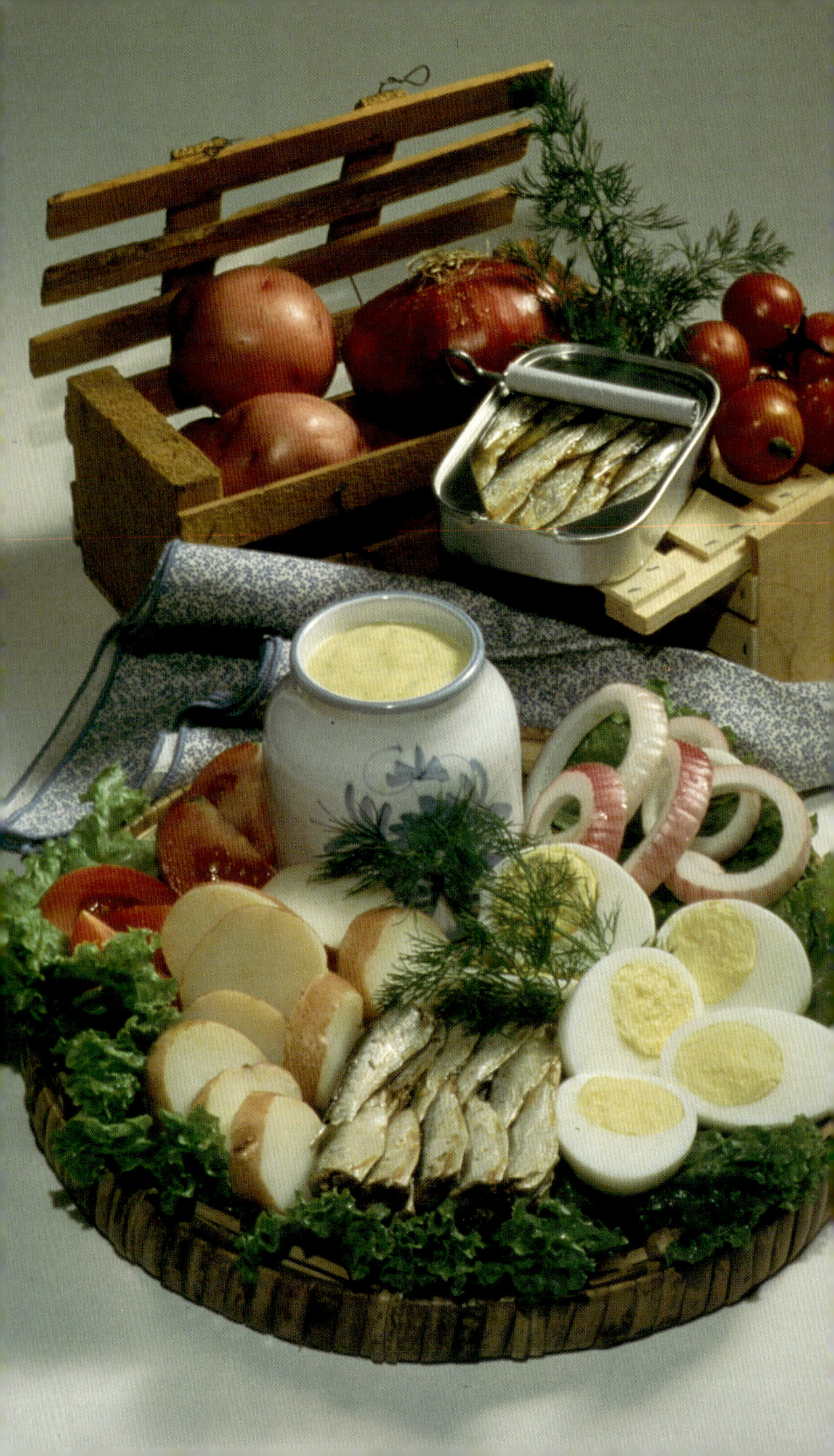

Viking Sardine Potato Salad

Makes 4 servings

Sardine-Mustard Sauce (recipe follows)

6 leaves red or green leaf lettuce

1 pound small red potatoes, cooked, cooled, and thickly sliced

4 hard-cooked eggs, halved

2 medium tomatoes, cut into wedges

1 medium red onion, sliced and separated into rings

3 cans (3.75 ounces each) Nordic brisling sardines in oil, drained

Dill sprigs (optional)

1. Prepare the Sardine Mustard Sauce; chill. Line a large platter with the lettuce leaves. Arrange the potatoes, eggs, tomatoes, onions, and remaining 2½ cans sardines on lettuce. Garnish with dill sprigs.
2. Drizzle several tablespoons of Sardine Mustard Sauce over salad. Pass the remaining dressing on the side.

Sardine Mustard Sauce

Makes about 1 cup

⅓ cup mayonnaise

⅓ cup sour cream

2 tablespoons prepared Dijon mustard

1 tablespoon prepared white horseradish

1 tablespoon fresh lemon juice

1 teaspoon dill weed

½ can of drained sardines, mashed with a fork

In a small bowl, combine all ingredients except sardines and blend until combined. Add sardines and blend well.

Norway Summer Rice Salad

MAKES 4 SERVINGS

1 head Boston lettuce, leaves washed and dried

3 cups cooked rice, chilled

Salt

1 medium cucumber, sliced

2 large carrots, shredded

1 bunch radishes, trimmed and halved

12 medium mushrooms, sliced

2 cans (3.75 ounces each) Nordic brisling sardines in oil, drained

¼ cup sliced scallions

Sesame Dressing (recipe follows)

Line a serving platter with the lettuce leaves. Season the rice with salt to taste and spoon it into the center of the lettuce leaves. Arrange the cucumbers, carrots, radishes, mushrooms, and sardines on lettuce surrounding rice. Sprinkle with sliced scallions. Serve with Sesame Dressing on the side.

Sesame Dressing

MAKES ABOUT 1 CUP

½ cup white vinegar

6 tablespoons extra-virgin olive oil

3 tablespoons soy sauce

1½ teaspoons dry mustard

3 tablespoons toasted sesame seeds

In a blender or mini food processor, combine all the ingredients. Blend until smooth, about 1 minute. Store refrigerated in a covered container for up to 1 week. Mix before serving.

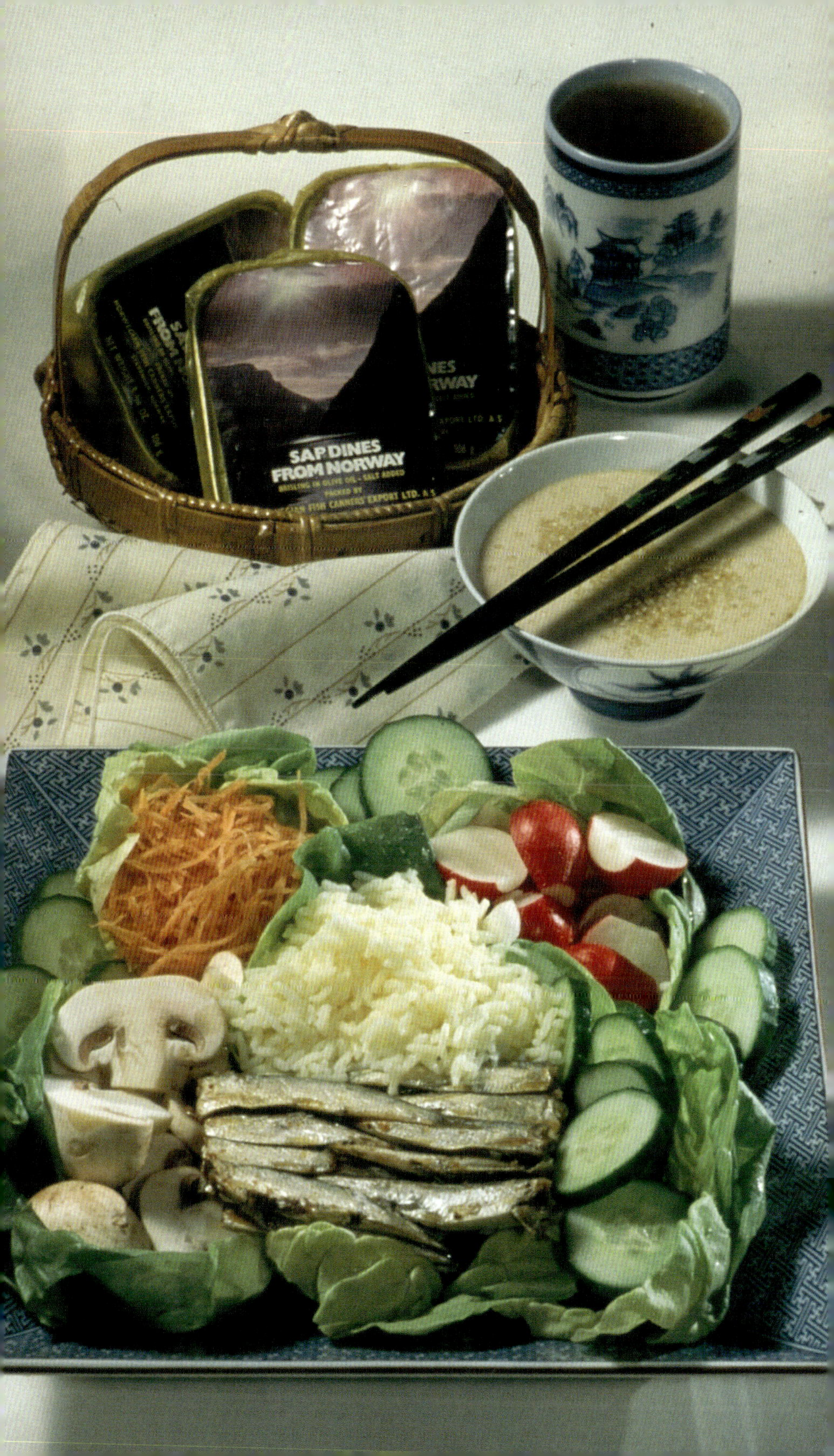
FROM NORWAY

East-West Sardine Salad

Makes 4 servings

Ginger-Chili Dressing (recipe follows)

2 ounces bean thread or cellophane noodles

Vegetable oil

2 cups thinly sliced celery

⅓ cup thinly sliced water chestnuts

1 medium red bell pepper, cut into thin strips

1 cup thinly sliced cucumber

1 cup thinly sliced mushrooms

2 cans (3.75 ounces each) Nordic brisling sardines in oil, drained

1. Make Ginger-Chili Dressing; set aside. In a 6-inch skillet, heat ¼-inch vegetable oil over medium-high heat until very hot. Cut uncooked noodles into 4 bundles. Add one-fourth of the noodles to the skillet and cook over high heat until puffed, about 30 seconds. Turn over and cook on the other side, about 30 seconds. Immediately transfer to paper towels to drain. Repeat with remaining noodles.
2. To serve, place a fried-noodle pancake on each of 4 plates. Top wit celery, water chestnuts, bell peppers, cucumbers, mushrooms, and sardines. Drizzle the dressing over the salads, dividing equally.

Ginger-Chili Dressing

6 tablespoons rice vinegar

1 tablespoon sugar

1½ tablespoons minced fresh ginger

¼ teaspoon crushed hot red pepper

5 tablespoons vegetable oil

1 tablespoon Asian sesame oil

Salt

In a small bowl, whisk together vinegar, sugar, ginger, and red pepper. In a second small bowl, combine the oils and whisk into vinegar mixture. Season with salt to taste.

Artichoke Gratin with Sardines

MAKES 4 SERVINGS

2 cans (3.75 ounces each) Nordic brisling sardines in oil, drained

3 tablespoons fresh lemon juice

3 tablespoons extra-virgin olive oil

2 packages (10 ounces each) frozen artichoke hearts, thawed

2 tablespoons finely chopped parsley

1 medium shallot, minced

Salt and freshly ground black pepper

⅓ cup whole-wheat bread crumbs

2 tablespoons grated Pecorino Romano cheese

1. Heat the oven to 375°F. Sprinkle the sardines with 1 tablespoon of the lemon juice.
2. Use 1 teaspoon of the olive oil to lightly oil a 12-inch oval gratin or small baking dish.
3. Arrange half the artichokes on the bottom of the dish. Sprinkle with half the parsley and shallot and season with salt and pepper. Arrange the sardines over the artichokes. Cover with the remaining artichokes. Sprinkle the remaining parsley and shallot over them and season again with salt and pepper.
4. In a small bowl, toss together the bread crumbs and cheese; sprinkle over the artichoke mixture. Drizzle with the remaining 2 tablespoons olive oil. Bake for 20 minutes or until the gratin is hot and the top is lightly browned.

Portuguese Stew with Sardines and Chorizo

Makes 3 servings

1 medium onion, finely chopped

3 tablespoons extra-virgin olive oil

4 cloves garlic, chopped

¼ pound chorizo sausage, thinly sliced

¾ pound Yukon Gold or red-skinned potatoes, peeled and cut into ¾-inch chunks

4 cups fat-free chicken broth

1 cup canned diced tomatoes

2 tablespoons chopped fresh parsley

2 teaspoons chopped fresh thyme leaves, or 1 teaspoon dried thyme

1 bay leaf

2 cans (3.75 ounces each) Nordic brisling sardines in oil, drained

Salt and freshly ground black pepper

1. In a medium-size stockpot or flameproof casserole dish, cook the onion in the olive oil over medium-low heat, covered, for 3 to 5 minutes, until softened.
2. Add the garlic and chorizo. Raise the heat to medium-high and cook 2 to 3 minutes longer, until the garlic is fragrant and the onion just begins to color.
3. Add the potatoes and stir to coat with the oil. Add the broth, tomatoes, half the parsley, the thyme, and bay leaf. Bring to a boil, reduce the heat to a slow boil, and cook until the potatoes are tender, 12 to 15 minutes.
4. Add the sardines and simmer 2 minutes longer. Remove and discard the bay leaf. Season the stew with salt and pepper to taste. Serve in soup plates. Garnish with the remaining chopped parsley.

Santa Fe Sardine and Olive Pasta

Makes 4 servings

3 tablespoons extra-virgin olive oil

3 cloves garlic, minced

1 medium red onion, sliced

½ cup pitted black olives, halved

1 cup corn kernels

1 cup medium or hot prepared chunky salsa

¼ cup chopped cilantro

2 tablespoons fresh lime juice

8 ounces pasta of your choice, cooked and drained

2 cans (3.75 ounces each) Nordic brisling sardines in oil, drained

1 avocado, peeled and cut into ½-inch chunks

Freshly grated Parmesan cheese

1. Heat olive oil in a large skillet over medium heat. Add garlic and onion; cook until onion is softened, about 3 minutes. Stir in the olives, corn, salsa, cilantro, and lime juice; reduce heat and simmer for 5 minutes.
2. Add the pasta and stir just until heated through. Transfer to a serving dish. Top with sardines and avocado chunks. Sprinkle with the Parmesan. Serve hot with additional Parmesan on the side.

Sweet Peppers Stuffed with Sardine Pasta Salad

MAKES 4 SERVINGS

3 cups cooked small pasta shells, cooled

1 cup shredded carrots

¼ cup sliced scallions

¼ cup Vinaigrette (see recipe page 87)

1½ tablespoons Dijon mustard

1½ tablespoons fresh lemon juice

½ teaspoon freshly ground pepper

2 cans (3.75 ounces each) Nordic brisling sardines in oil, drained

Salt

4 large green or red bell peppers

1. In a large bowl, combine the pasta, carrots, and scallions. In a small bowl, blend the mayonnaise, mustard, lemon juice, and pepper; stir into the pasta mixture. Add to sardines and toss gently to mix. Season with salt to taste.
2. Slice the tops off the peppers; reserve tops. Remove the seeds and membranes from the peppers. Fill each pepper with sardine mixture, dividing equally and packing lightly. Replace the tops and wrap each pepper snugly in plastic wrap. Refrigerate until ready to serve.

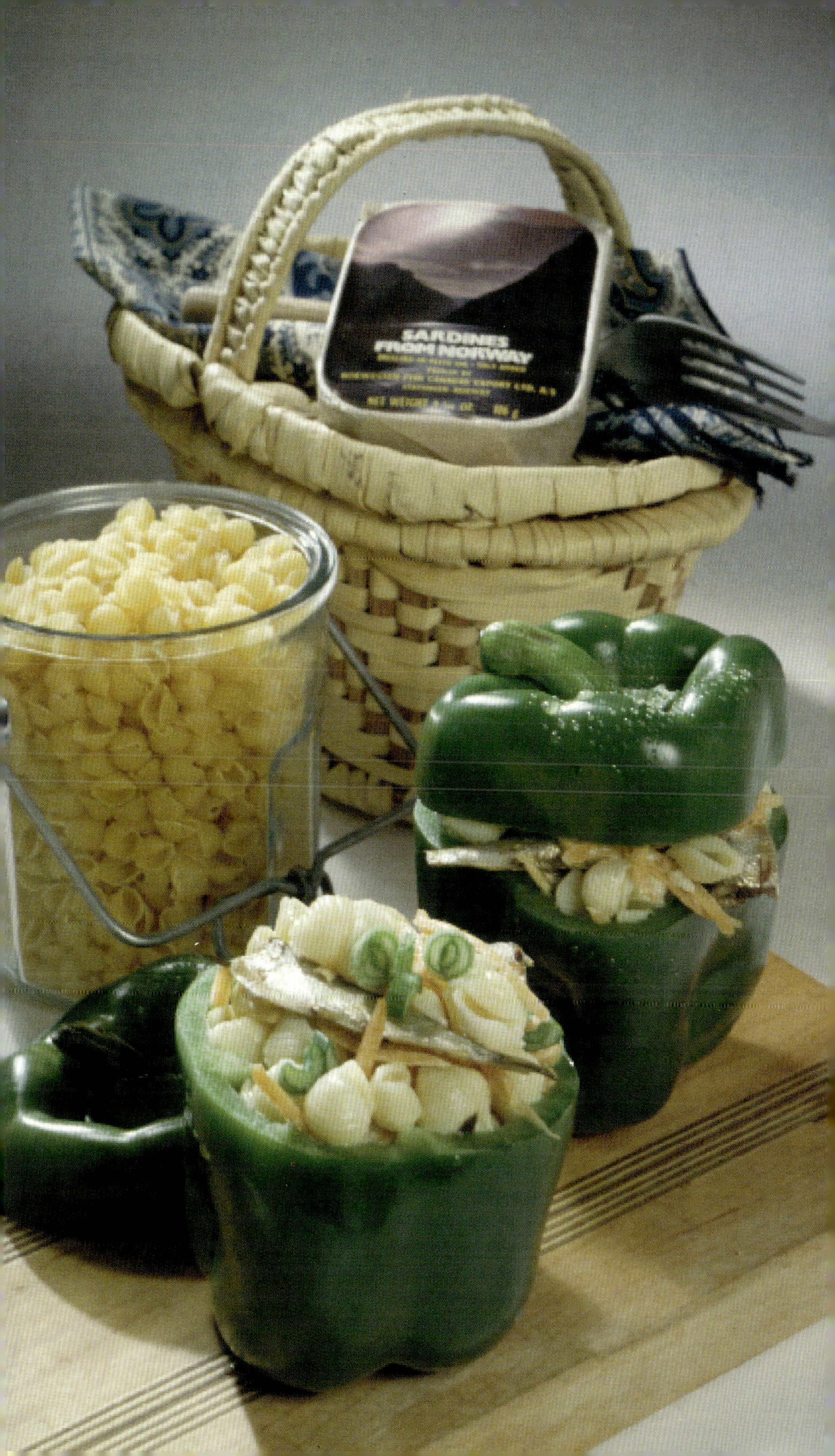
SARDINES
FROM NORWAY

Recipe Index